Memory: A Very Short Introduction

VERY SHORT INTRODUCTIONS are for anyone wanting a stimulating and accessible way into a new subject. They are written by experts, and have been translated into more than 45 different languages.

The series began in 1995, and now covers a wide variety of topics in every discipline. The VSI library now contains over 500 volumes—a Very Short Introduction to everything from Psychology and Philosophy of Science to American History and Relativity—and continues to grow in every subject area.

Titles in the series include the following:

Jonathan K. Foster

MEMORY

A Very Short Introduction

OXFORD
UNIVERSITY PRESS

OXFORD
UNIVERSITY PRESS

Great Clarendon Street, Oxford OX2 6DP

Oxford University Press is a department of the University of Oxford.
It furthers the University's objective of excellence in research, scholarship,
and education by publishing worldwide in

Oxford New York

Auckland Cape Town Dar es Salaam Hong Kong Karachi
Kuala Lumpur Madrid Melbourne Mexico City Nairobi
New Delhi Shanghai Taipei Toronto

With offices in

Argentina Austria Brazil Chile Czech Republic France Greece
Guatemala Hungary Italy Japan Poland Portugal Singapore
South Korea Switzerland Thailand Turkey Ukraine Vietnam

Oxford is a registered trade mark of Oxford University Press
in the UK and in certain other countries

Published in the United States
by Oxford University Press Inc., New York

British Library Cataloguing in Publication Data

Data available

Library of Congress Cataloging in Publication Data

Data available

ISBN 978-0-19-280675-8

Typeset by SPI Publisher Services, Pondicherry, India
Printed and bound by CPI Group (UK) Ltd, Croydon, CR0 4YY

Contents

List of illustrations

The publisher and the author apologize for any errors or omissions in the above list. If contacted they will be pleased to rectify these at the earliest opportunity.

Chapter 1
You are your memory

There seems something more speakingly incomprehensible in the powers, the failures, the inequalities of memory, than in any other of our intelligences.

Jane Austen

This chapter will emphasize how important memory is for virtually everything that we do. Without it, we would be unable to speak, read, identify objects, navigate our way around our environment, or maintain personal relationships. To illustrate this point, some anecdotal observations and considerations of memory will be offered, together with observations made by important thinkers in other, related fields such as literature and philosophy. We then consider a brief history of systematic, scientific investigations into memory, which began with Ebbinghaus in the late 19th century and then progressed via Bartlett in the 1930s to controlled, group-based experimental research conducted in the context of recent information-processing models of memory. We conclude by considering how we study memory today, and the principles of good design in contemporary memory research.

The importance of memory

> Why should this absolutely God-given faculty retain so much better
> the events of yesterday than those of last year, and, best of all, those
> of an hour ago? Why, again, in old age should its grasp of
> childhood's events seem firmest? Why should repeating an
> experience strengthen our recollection of it? Why should drugs,
> fevers, asphyxia, and excitement resuscitate things long since
> forgotten? . . . such peculiarities seem quite fantastic; and might, for
> aught we can see *a priori*, be the precise opposites of what they are.
> Evidently, then, the faculty does not exist absolutely, but works
> under conditions; and the quest of the conditions becomes the
> psychologist's most interesting task.
>
> William James (1890), quoted in
> *Principles of Psychology*, i. 3

In the quote above, William James mentions some of the many
intriguing aspects of memory. In this chapter, we will touch on
some of its fascinating features. However, in a chapter of this
length and scope we will, of course, only really be able to scratch
the surface of what has been one of the most thoroughly
researched areas of psychological enquiry.

The reason for the range of work that has been conducted into
the questions of what, why, and how we remember should be
apparent: memory is a key psychological process. As stated by the
eminent cognitive neuroscientist Michel Gazzaniga: 'Everything in
life is memory, save for the thin edge of the present'. Memory
allows us to recall birthdays, holidays, and other significant events
that may have taken place hours, days, months, or even many
years ago. Our memories are personal and 'internal', yet without
memory we wouldn't be able to undertake 'external' acts – such
as holding a conversation, recognizing our friends' faces,
remembering appointments, acting on new ideas, succeeding
at work, or even learning to walk.

Memory in everyday life

Memory is far more than simply bringing to mind information encountered at some previous time. Whenever the experience of some past event influences someone at a later time, the influence of the previous experience is a reflection of memory for that past event.

The vagaries of memory can be illustrated by the following example. Without doubt, you have seen thousands of coins in your lifetime. But let us reflect on how well you can remember a typical coin that you may have in your pocket. Without looking at it, take a few minutes to try to draw a coin of a particular denomination from memory. Now compare your drawing with the coin itself. How accurate was your memory for the coin? For instance, was the head facing the correct way? How many of the words (if any!) from the coin did you recall? Did you place these words correctly?

Systematic studies were conducted into this very topic in the 1970s and 1980s. Researchers found that, in fact, most people have very poor memories for very familiar things – like coins. This represents a type of memory which we tend to take for granted (but which – in a sense – doesn't really exist!). Try it with other familiar objects in your environment, such as stamps, or try to remember the details of clothes that other people in your workplace or with whom you frequently socialize typically wear. The key point here is that we tend to remember the information that is most salient and useful for us. For instance, we may be much better at recalling the typical size, dimensions or colour of coins than the direction of the head or the text on the coin, because the size, dimensions or colour may well be more relevant for us when we are using money (i.e. for the primary purpose of payment and exchange for which money was devised). And when remembering people, we will typically recall their faces and other distinguishing features that remain relatively invariant (and are, therefore, most useful in identifying them), rather than items which may change (such as individuals' clothing).

Instead of thinking of coins and clothing, it is perhaps more straightforward for most people to consider the role of memory in the case of a student who i) attends a lecture, and ii) later brings to mind successfully what was taught in the lecture in the examination hall. This is the type of 'memory' that we are all familiar with from our own school days. But it may be less obvious that memory may still play an effective role for the student, even when the person does not 'remember' the lecture or the information *per se*, but instead uses information from the lecture more generally (i.e. possibly without thinking about the lecture itself – or recalling the specific information that was presented in that context; this is termed *episodic memory*).

In the case of the student's more general use of the information presented in the lecture, we refer to this information as having entered *semantic memory*, which is broadly analogous with what we also refer to as 'general knowledge'. Furthermore, if that student later develops an interest (or a marked disinterest) in the topic of the lecture, this interest may itself reflect memory for the earlier lecture, even though the student might not be able to recall consciously having ever attended a lecture on the topic in question.

Similarly, memory plays a role whether or not we intend to learn. In fact, comparatively little of our time is spent trying to 'record' events for later remembering, as in formal study. By contrast, most of the time we are simply getting on with our everyday lives. But if, in this everyday life, something salient happens (which, in our evolutionary past as *homo sapiens*, may well have been associated with threat or reward), then established physiological and psychological processes kick in, and we usually remember these events quite well. For example, most of us have had the experience

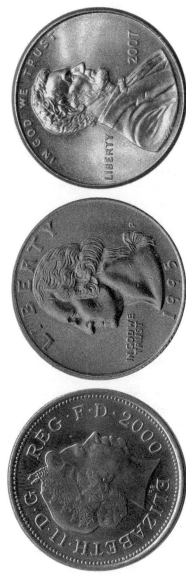

1. Our memory for very familiar objects – like coins – is typically considerably worse than we believe to be the case

of forgetting where we left our car in a large car park. But if we have an accident while parking and damage our car and/or the car of our neighbour in the car park, then specific 'fight, fright or flight' mechanisms are initiated, ensuring that we typically remember such events (and the location of our car) very well!

So memory is not, in fact, dependent upon an intention to remember events. Furthermore, past events only have to influence our *thoughts*, *feelings*, or *behaviour* (as we considered with the earlier example of the student attending the lecture) for this to provide sufficient evidence of our memory for these events. Memory also plays a role regardless of our intention to retrieve or utilize past events. Many of the influences of past events are unintended, and may 'pop into mind' unexpectedly. Retrieval of information may even run counter to our intentions, as shown in work conducted by researchers over the past several decades. This issue has become very topical of late in the context of phenomena such as the retrieval of traumatic memories.

Models and mechanisms of memory

There have been many different models of how memory works, going right back into classical times. For example, Plato regarded memory as being like a wax tablet, on which impressions would be made or *encoded*, and subsequently *stored*, so that we could return to and *retrieve* these impressions (i.e. memories) at a later time. This tripartite distinction between *encoding*, *storage* and *retrieval* has persisted among scientific investigators to the present day. Other philosophers in classical times likened memories to birds in an aviary or to books in a library, underlining the difficulties of retrieving information after it had been stored – that is, catching the right bird or locating the right book.

Contemporary theorists have come to appreciate that memory is a *selective* and *interpretive* process. In other words, there is more to memory than just the passive storage of information.

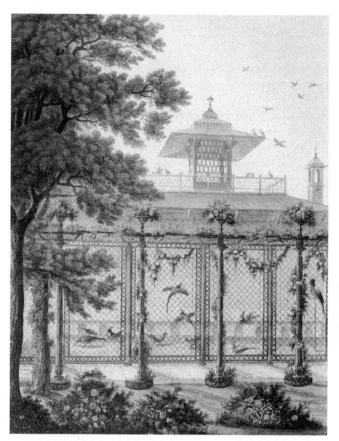

2. Bird in an aviary – retrieving the correct memory has sometimes been compared to catching the correct bird in an aviary full of birds

Furthermore, after learning and storing new information, we can select, interpret and integrate one thing with another – so as to make better use of what we learn and remember. This is likely to be one reason why chess experts find it easier to remember the position of pieces on a chess board, and why football fans find it easier to remember each of the football scores at the weekend,

7

i.e. thanks to their extensive knowledge and the interconnections between different elements of this knowledge.

At the same time, our memory is far from perfect. As encapsulated by the writer and philosopher C. S. Lewis:

> Five senses; an incurably abstract intellect; a haphazardly selective memory; a set of preconceptions and assumptions so numerous that I can never examine more than minority of them – never become conscious of them all. How much of total reality can such an apparatus let through?

Yet, there are things that we need to remember in order to function effectively in the world, and other things that we do not need to remember. As we have already noted, the things that we need to remember often have evolutionary significance: in situations of 'threat' or 'reward' (either actual or perceived), cognitive and brain mechanisms are invoked that help us to remember better.

Thinking along these lines has led many contemporary researchers to regard the *mechanisms underlying memory as being best characterized as a dynamic activity* or *process* rather than as a *static entity* or *thing*.

The Ebbinghaus tradition

Although personal observations and anecdotes about memory can be illuminating and entertaining, they often originate from a specific experience of a given individual. It is therefore open to question to what degree they are a) objectively 'real' and b) can be generalized universally, to all individuals. Systematic scientific research can offer unique insight into these issues. Some of the classic systematic research in memory and forgetting was conducted in the late 19th century by Hermann Ebbinghaus. Ebbinghaus taught himself 169 separate lists of 13 nonsense syllables. Each syllable comprised a 'meaningless' consonant-vowel-consonant trigram (e.g. PEL). Ebbinghaus relearned each of these lists after an interval ranging from 21 minutes to 31 days. He was especially interested in the extent to which forgetting had occurred over this time period, using the 'savings score' (i.e. how much time it took him to relearn the list) as a measure of how much he had forgotten.

Ebbinghaus noted that the rate of forgetting was roughly exponential: that is, forgetting is rapid at first (soon after the material has been learned), but the rate at which information is forgotten gradually decreases. So the rate of forgetting is logarithmic rather than linear. This observation has stood the test of time well, and has been shown to apply across a range of different materials and learning conditions. So, if you stop studying the French language after you leave school, in the first 12 months you will show a rapid decline in your French vocabulary. But the rate at which you forget this vocabulary will gradually slow down over time. So that, if you study French again five or ten years later, you might be surprised at how much you have actually retained (compared with how much you remembered a few years earlier).

Another interesting feature of memory noted by Ebbinghaus is that, having 'lost' information such as some of your French vocabulary, you can relearn this information much faster than someone who has never learned French in the first place (i.e. the concept of 'savings'). This finding implies that there must be a residual trace of this 'lost' information in your brain. This point also attests to the important issue regarding *conscious* versus *unconscious* knowledge that we will consider in later chapters: we are obviously not conscious of this 'lost' French vocabulary, but the research findings regarding this preserved information indicate that there must be some retention of the memory record at an unconscious level. A closely related point is made by the eminent psychologist B.F. Skinner when he writes that

'Education is what survives when what has been learnt has been forgotten.' We might add '... consciously forgotten but retained in some other residual form'.

Ebbinghaus' classic work in the field, *On Memory*, was published in 1885. This work encompasses Ebbinghaus' many enduring contributions to memory research, including the nonsense syllable, the identification of exponential forgetting and the concept of savings (plus the several memory problems Ebbinghaus worked on systematically in his research, such as the effects of repetition, the shape of the forgetting curve, and the comparison of poetry and nonsense-syllable learning). The great advantage of the experimental methodology practised by Ebbinghaus is that it controls for a lot of extraneous (and potentially distorting) factors that may influence memory. Ebbinghaus described his nonsense syllables as being 'uniformly unassociated' – which he regarded as

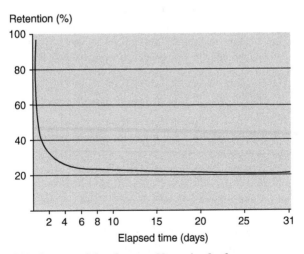

3. Ebbinghaus noted that the rate of forgetting for the consonant-vowel-consonant trigrams that he taught himself was roughly exponential (i.e. forgetting was rapid at first, but the rate at which information was forgotten gradually decreased)

a strength of his approach. But he could be criticized for failing to use more meaningful memory materials. Some workers in the field have argued that Ebbinghaus' approach tends to oversimplify memory, reducing its subtleties to a series of artificial, mathematical components. The risk from such an approach is that – although we are employing scientific rigour, and are able to partition the mechanisms of memory into tractable chunks – we may be eliminating those very aspects of human memory that are most intrinsic to (and definitive of) the way our memory functions in everyday life. An important question therefore concerns the following: to what extent are Ebbinghaus' findings generalizable to human memory as a whole?

The Bartlett tradition

The second great tradition in memory research is exemplified by the work of Frederick Bartlett, conducted in the first half of the 20th century – i.e. several decades after Ebbinghaus. In his book *Remembering*, published in 1932, Bartlett challenged the Ebbinghaus tradition, which at the time was pre-eminent in the field. Bartlett argued that the study of nonsense syllables doesn't tell us much about the way human memory operates in the real world. He raised an important question: how many people spend their lives remembering nonsense syllables? In contrast to Ebbinghaus, who tried to eliminate meaning from his test materials, Bartlett focused on the very opposite – meaningful materials (more specifically, materials on which we try to impose some meaning). These materials were learned and remembered by Bartlett's participants under relatively naturalistic conditions. Indeed, it appears to be a fundamental element of the 'human condition' that, in our natural state, we do typically seek to impose meaning upon events taking place in our environment. This principle is underscored by much of Bartlett's work. For example, in some of Bartlett's most influential studies, subjects were asked to read a story to themselves (the most famous story being 'The War of the Ghosts'); they then tried to recall the story later.

Bartlett found that individuals recalled each story in their own idiosyncratic way, but he also discovered some general trends among his findings:

- the stories tended to become shorter when they were remembered;
- the stories also became more coherent: i.e. people seemed to make sense of unfamiliar material by linking this material to their pre-existing ideas, general knowledge and cultural expectations;
- the changes people made when remembering a story tended to be associated with the reactions and emotions they experienced when they first heard it.

Bartlett argued that what people remember is, to some extent, mediated by their emotional and personal commitment to – and investment in – the original to-be-remembered event. In Bartlett's own words, memory retains 'a little outstanding detail', while the remainder of what we remember represents an elaboration that is merely influenced by the original event. Bartlett referred to this key characteristic of memory as 'reconstructive', as opposed to 'reproductive'. In other words, instead of *reproducing* the original event or story, we derive a *reconstruction* based on our existing presuppositions, expectations and our 'mental set'.

As an example, think of the way two people supporting two different countries (England and Germany) report the events in a football match they have just watched (the England football team playing against Germany's football team). The same objective events took place on the playing field, but the England supporter will most likely report the events in a markedly different way from the supporter of the German team. And when two people see the same film, their reported memories of the film will be similar, but there will typically be significant differences as well. Why might their reports be different? This will depend on their interests, motivations and emotional reaction – how they apprehend the presented narrative. Likewise, someone who voted for the current government in the last general election may well remember events pertaining to a major national event (a war, for instance) in quite a different way from someone who voted for the current opposition party. (These examples also hint at the manner in which social factors – including stereotypes – can influence our memory of events.)

There is, therefore, a crucial difference in the approach to memory that was taken by Ebbinghaus and Bartlett. The essence of Bartlett's argument is that people attempt to impose meaning on what they observe in the world, and that this influences their memory for events. This may not be important in a laboratory experiment using relatively abstract, meaningless materials, such as the nonsense syllables employed by Ebbinghaus. But Bartlett argued that, in a more naturalistic setting, this *effort after meaning* is one of the most significant features of the way our memory works in the real world.

Constructing memory

As we have seen from the work of Bartlett, memory is not a veridical copy of the world, unlike a DVD or video recording. It is perhaps more helpful to think of memory as an influence of the world on the individual. Indeed, a *constructivist approach* describes memory as the combined influences of the world and the person's own ideas and expectations. For example, the experience of each person while they are watching a film will be somewhat different because they are different individuals, drawing upon different personal pasts, and with different values, thoughts, goals, feelings, expectations, moods and past experiences. They might have been seated next to one another in the cinema, but in an important sense they actually experienced subjectively different films. So an event, as it occurs, is constructed by the person who experienced it. This construction is greatly influenced by the memory 'event' (in this case, the film screening), but it is also a product of each person's individual characteristics and personal idiosyncrasies (all of which play a substantial role in how the event is experienced, *encoded* and subsequently *stored*).

Later, when we come to try to remember that event, some parts of the film come readily to mind, whereas other parts we may re-construct – based on the parts that we remember and on what we know or believe must have happened. (The latter is likely to be predicated on our inferential processes about the world, combined with the elements of the film that we recall.) In fact, we are so good at this sort of re-construction (or 'filling in the gaps') that we are often consciously unaware that it has happened. This seems especially likely to happen when a memory is told and retold, with different influences present at each time of retrieval (see the reference to Bartlett's techniques of serial and repeated reproduction cited in the box on page 15). In such situations, the 're-constructed' memory often seems as real as the 'recollected' memory. This is an especially worrying consideration when we reflect on the degree to which people can feel that they are 'remembering' crucial features of a witnessed murder or a personally experienced childhood assault, when – instead – they may be 're-constructing' these events and filling in missing information based on their general knowledge of the world (see Chapter 4).

In the light of these considerations, the act of remembering has been likened to the task of a paleontologist who constructs a dinosaur from an incomplete set of bones, but who possesses a great deal of general knowledge about dinosaurs. In this analogy, the past event leaves us with access to an incomplete set of bones (with occasional 'foreign' bones that are not derived from the past event at all). Our knowledge of the world then influences our efforts to re-assemble those bones into something that resembles the past episode. The memory that we assemble may contain some actual elements of the past (i.e. some real bones), but – taken as a whole – it is an imperfect re-construction of the past located in the present.

The War of the Ghosts

When Bartlett followed Ebbinghaus's lead and tried to carry out further experiments using nonsense syllables, the result was, so he reported, 'disappointment and a growing dissatisfaction'. Instead, he chose to work with ordinary prose material that 'would prove interesting in itself' – the kind of material that Ebbinghaus had, in fact, rejected.

Bartlett used two basic methods in his experiments:
Serial reproduction, similar to the game of 'Chinese Whispers'. One person passes some information to a second person, who then passes the same information to a third, and so on. The 'story' that reaches the final person in the group is then compared with the original.

Repeated reproduction is where someone is asked to repeat the same piece of information at certain intervals (from 15 minutes to a few years) after first learning it.

The most famous piece of prose Bartlett used to investigate recall is a North American folktale called *The War of the Ghosts*:

One night two young men from Egulac went down to the river to hunt seals, and while they were there it became foggy and calm. Then they heard war cries, and they thought: 'Maybe this is a war-party.' They escaped to the shore, and hid behind a log. Now canoes came up, and they heard the noise of paddles, and saw one canoe coming up to them. There were five men in the canoe, and they said:

'What do you think? We wish to take you along. We are going up the river to make war on the people.' One of the young men said: 'I have no arrows.' 'Arrows are in the canoe,' they said. 'I will not go along. I might be killed. My relatives do not know where I have gone. But you,' he said, turning to the other, 'may go with them.' So one of the young men went, but the other returned home.

And the warriors went on up the river to a town on the other side of Kalama. The people came down to the water, and they began to fight, and many were killed. But presently the young man heard one of the warriors say: 'Quick, let us go home: that Indian has been hit.' Now he thought: 'Oh, they are ghosts.' He did not feel sick, but they said he had been shot.

So the canoes went back to Egulac, and the young man went ashore to his house, and made a fire. And he told everybody and said: 'Behold I accompanied the ghosts, and we went to fight. Many of our fellows were killed, and many of those who attacked us were killed. They said I was hit, and I did not feel sick.'

He told it all, and then he became quiet. When the sun rose he fell down. Something black came out of his mouth. His face became contorted. The people jumped up and cried. He was dead.

Bartlett chose this story because it does not relate to the English narrative culture of his participants, and appears to be disjointed and somewhat incoherent to Anglo-Saxon ears. Bartlett anticipated that these features of the story would exaggerate the transformation as his participants attempted to reproduce it.

As an example, here is one attempt by someone repeating the story for the fourth time, this time several months after first hearing it:

Two youths went down to the river to hunt for seals. They were hiding behind a rock when a boat with some warriors in it came up to them. The warriors, however, said they were friends, and invited them to help them to fight an enemy over the river. The elder one said he could not go because his relations would be so anxious if he did not return home. So the younger one went with the warriors in the boat.

In the evening he returned and told his friends that he had been fighting in a great battle, and that many were slain on both sides. After lighting a fire he retired to sleep. In the morning, when the sun rose, he fell ill, and his neighbours came to see him. He had told them that he had been wounded in the battle but had felt no pain then. But soon he became worse. He writhed and shrieked and fell to the ground dead. Something black came out of his mouth. The neighbours said he must have been at war with the ghosts.

From his experiments, Bartlett concluded that people tend to rationalize material that they are remembering. In other words, they try to make it easier to understand the material, and modify it into something they feel more comfortable with. Bartlett's own description of what was happening is as follows:

Remembering is not the re-excitation of innumerable fixed, lifeless and fragmentary traces. It is an imaginative reconstruction, or construction, built out of the relation of our attitude towards a whole active mass of organised past reactions or experience, and to a little outstanding detail which commonly appears in image or in language form. It is thus hardly ever really exact, even in the most rudimentary cases of rote recapitulation...

In this context, it is perhaps not surprising that people often find their memories to be somewhat unreliable, or that the accounts of two different people who have observed the same event may be somewhat different.

After considering two of the most influential figures in experimental memory research, we now turn to a consideration of more contemporary methods and findings.

How we study memory today

Memory can be studied in many ways and in many situations. It can be manipulated and studied in the 'real world'. However, most objective research on the topic of memory conducted to date has comprised experimental work, in which different manipulations are compared under controlled conditions (typically, in a laboratory setting) involving a set of to-be-remembered words or other similar materials. The manipulation might include any variable that is expected to influence memory, such as the nature of the material (e.g. visual vs. verbal stimuli), the familiarity of the material, the degree of similarity between study and test conditions, and the level of motivation to learn. Traditionally, experimental researchers have studied memory for the following types of stimuli: lists of words, non-word stimuli such as those used by Ebbinghaus, and other commonly available materials such as numbers or pictures (other sorts of materials have been used too; including texts, stories, poems, appointments and life events).

Over recent decades, much of the empirical research into memory that has been conducted has typically been interpreted in the context of information processing and computer models of memory that were adopted by most experimentalists after the Second World War. Within this framework, the functional properties underlying human memory (and other aspects of cognitive functioning) are considered broadly to reflect the type of information processing embodied by the modern computer. (Note that this metaphor typically refers to the functional properties or *software* of the computer, rather than to its *hardware*.) More recent research studies typically involve larger numbers of participants than were tested in the earlier work conducted by Ebbinghaus and Bartlett – who often focused on detailed examination of individual cases (including – in Ebbinghaus' case – himself!). Findings from group studies can be analysed using powerful inferential statistical techniques which enable us to interpret objectively the size and significance of the findings obtained.

Observation and inference: Memory research in the modern era

Memory is evident to the degree that an event influences later behaviour. But how can we know whether the later behaviour was influenced by the past event? In the final section of this chapter, we consider some of the techniques used by contemporary memory researchers.

Try this: write down the first 15 items of furniture that come to mind. Then compare your list to that on page 23. There are probably several matches. If you had studied a list of items of furniture names, and you had later been asked to remember them, could it be logically inferred that your listing of a given furniture item was directly attributable to your memory for the items on the previously presented list? This is not a valid inference: some items you might consciously recall as being from the previous list, other items you might think of due to an indirect or unconscious influence from studying the previous list, while some items you might think of just because they are items of furniture (i.e. not as a result of studying the word list at all). So it cannot necessarily be concluded that the number of matches between your list and the study list is a good measure of your memory for the list (because the matches might occur for any of the reasons mentioned in the last sentence).

This demonstration with the furniture list captures an important issue in memory research. As we have already noted, memory is not observed directly (unlike, say, a thunderstorm or a chemical reaction) – rather, it is inferred from a change in behaviour, typically measured via an observed change in performance on a task that is designed to measure memory. But performance on such a task will be influenced by other factors (such as one's motivation, interest, general knowledge, and associated reasoning processes), as well as being influenced by one's memory for the original event. So it is very important to be careful about what is i) *observed* (typically influenced by factors other than memory *per se*) and what is ii) *inferred* when conducting systematic research into the functional properties of memory.

To address this problem, memory research is typically conducted by comparing different groups of participants (or different manipulations of memory), organized such that the 'past event' or manipulation occurs for one group, but not for the others. The groups of participants are chosen so as to be equivalent (or at least very similar) on all potentially relevant dimensions; for example, groups will typically not differ in age, education or intelligence. This type of research design is the basis for most (if not all) of the material discussed in this book. The logical sequence is as follows: because the only known, relevant difference between groups of participants is the presence or absence of the memory event or manipulation, differences observed between groups at a later time are then assumed to reflect memory for that event. But it is important to note that this is an assumption (albeit, typically, a reasonable one); furthermore, it is essential to determine that there are no other differences between the groups of individuals being evaluated that could affect the outcome of the memory investigation.

Here is one such example of this approach, taken from the systematic investigation of the proposed phenomenon of 'sleep learning'. Suppose that you played tapes of information to yourself in your sleep, with the hope or expectation that you would remember the information later. How would you evaluate if these tapes were effective? To answer the question, you might present some information to people while they are sleep, then wake them up, and observe whether their subsequent behaviour reflected any memory for the information that was presented to them while they were asleep. Wood, Bootzin, Kihlstrom, and Schacter conducted an experiment that did this. While people slept, these researchers read out pairs of category names and member names (e.g. 'a metal: gold'). Each pair of *category: item* word pairs was repeated several times. After ten minutes, the participants in the study who had been asleep during stimulus presentation were woken up, and asked to generate exemplars from named categories (such as metals) as they came to mind. The assumption underlying this study was that, if participants remembered having the words read to them while they slept, then they would be more likely to include gold in the list of metal names that they subsequently generated.

However (as per the considerations that were mentioned previously), to make a valid inference about the remembered information, it is clearly not enough to observe how often exemplars that had been presented while the participants were asleep appeared in the subsequently generated lists. For example, many people – when asked to think of metals – would include gold, even without it having been previously read to them while they slept. According to the principles of good research design mentioned earlier, researchers can overcome this type of problem by examining the difference between the performance of a matched group or comparison condition with that of an experimental group or condition.

In their study, Wood and colleagues made two comparisons. The first comparison was between groups: some participants were awake while the word pairs were read to them, while some were asleep. Because matched participants were randomly assigned to the 'sleep' or 'awake' groups, comparing how often the target words appeared in each of these two groups showed whether people were more influenced by i) presentations while they were awake or by ii) presentations while they were asleep. Indeed, in this study people who were awake during the paired presentations were more than twice as likely to report the target exemplars, compared with people who had slept during the paired presentations. This particular comparison shows (perhaps unsurprisingly) that learning while awake is better than learning while asleep. However, note that this comparison does not rule out the possibility that the memory performance of those who had slept was beneficially influenced by the previous paired presentations of *category: item* words.

The researchers therefore made another important comparison, which involved repeating their measures quite cleverly. There were actually two different lists of word pairs used in the study – one list included 'a metal: gold' while the other list included 'a flower: pansy'. Each participant was read only one of the lists of paired words while asleep, but *all* participants were tested on *both* category lists after being woken. This procedure allowed the experimenters to compare how often people, after being woken, produced category exemplars that had been read to them compared to exemplars that had not been read to them. In other words, multiple observations were made for each participant in the study, and then compared.

When this comparison was made in those individuals who had heard some of the *category: item* pairs while they were asleep, the findings indicated that there was no real difference between individuals' subsequent reports of key category exemplars a) when the exemplars had previously been read to them compared with b) when the exemplars had not been read to them. By contrast, if people were awake during word presentation, an analogous comparison between a) and b) showed that the presentations of the lists had a significant effect on subsequent memory for the key exemplars.

Summary

We have noted in this chapter that memory is essential for virtually everything that we do. Without it, we would be unable to speak, read, navigate our way around our environment, identify objects or maintain interpersonal relationships. Although personal observations and anecdotes about memory can be illuminating and entertaining, they often originate from a specific experience of a given individuals. It is therefore questionable to what degree such observations can be generalized universally, i.e. to all individuals. We have seen from the work of Ebbinghaus and Bartlett how systematic research can provide crucial insight into the functional properties of human memory. More recently, it has been possible to analyse the functional properties underlying memory systematically using powerful observational and statistical techniques that enable us to interpret the size and significance of findings obtained from carefully controlled experiments. The following chapters of this book will consider some of the most salient findings obtained from such studies. As we will see, it is more accurate to regard our memory as an *activity* rather than as a *thing*. Furthermore, one of the most important aspects of recent scientific discoveries is that, rather than being perceived as a single entity ('my memory' this ... or 'my memory' that ...), we now know that memory represents a collection of several different capacities. This issue will be addressed further in Chapter 2.

Furniture list (from page 19)

Chair	Wardrobe
Table	Bookcase
Stool	Desk
Cupboard	Cabinet
Bed	Closet
Sofa	Chest

Chapter 2
Mapping memories

This section of the book will consider the central question of how memory systems operate, and how different functional memory components may be defined. The central point will be made that any memory system, whether it be the human brain (sometimes referred to as the 'most complex system in the known universe'), the hard disk of a PC, a video recorder, or a humble office filing cabinet, needs to be able to i) encode, ii) store, and iii) retrieve information effectively if it is to function well as a memory system. Memory can fail if there are difficulties with any of these three processes. Having discussed this point, I will next turn to a consideration of the ways in which different component processes within memory have been defined. I here argue that our personal impressions of having either a good memory or a poor memory (in the singular) are incorrect. By contrast, much research conducted over the past 100 years in both healthy participants and in brain injured clinical patients has illustrated the manner in which memory separates into multiple, distinct components. The key distinction between a) short-term and b) long-term memory (often misunderstood both by clinicians and by the lay community alike) will be made using appropriate analogies. Different functional elements within short-term and long-term memory will then be considered. This chapter will provide a conceptual framework within which much of the material presented in the remainder of this book can be understood.

The logic of memory: encoding, storage, and retrieval

There's rosemary, that's for remembrance; pray, love, remember

Shakespeare, Hamlet

Any effective memory system – whether it's an audio- or videocassette recorder, the hard disk of your computer or even a simple filing cabinet – needs to do three things well. It has to be able to:

1. *encode* (i.e. take in or acquire) information,
2. *store* or retain that information faithfully and, in the case of long-term memory, over a significant period of time,
3. *retrieve* or access that stored information.

So, using the filing cabinet analogy, first you file a document in a particular location. The document is then held in that location, and when you need it you go to retrieve it from the filing cabinet. But unless you have a good search system, you're not going to be able to find the document easily. So memory involves not just taking in and storing information, but the ability to retrieve it too. And all three components have to work well together if our memory is to work efficiently.

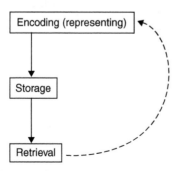

4. The logical distinction between encoding, storage, and retrieval is central when we are considering the operation of human memory

Problems in encoding are often related to poor attention, whereas difficulties in storage are what we refer to in everyday speech as forgetting. With retrieval, an important distinction is often made between *availability* and *accessibility*. For example, sometimes we can't quite recall someone's name, but it feels as if it's right on the tip of our tongue. We may know the first letter of the name, and the number of syllables, but we just can't produce the word itself. Not surprisingly, this is called the 'tip of the tongue phenomenon'. We know we have the information stored somewhere, and we may have partial knowledge of it (so the information is, in theory, available), but it's not currently accessible. One has an enormous amount of information stored in one's memory that is potentially available at any given moment, but there is typically only a small portion of information available for access at any given time.

Memory can fail to work due to a blockage in any one, or more, of these three components (*encoding*, *storage*, and *retrieval*). In the tip of the tongue phenomenon example, it's the retrieval component that's failing. All three components are necessary for effective memory, but no one component is sufficient: this is the fundamental logic of memory.

Different kinds of memory: the functional structure of remembering

Plato and his contemporaries based their speculations about the mind on their own personal impressions. This still happens today – especially among some people who dismiss systematic findings about the brain and mind as 'just common sense'. But we now have experimental (often called *empirical*) information on which to base our theories. We conduct rigorous, highly controlled experimental studies to collect objective information about the workings of human memory (see Chapter 1). And, as we shall see, several of these well-established findings contradict the 'common sense' relied on by many people.

Experimenters have applied a number of systematic techniques in their efforts to understand memory. One approach has been to subdivide the vast field of memory into areas that seem to function differently from each another. Think about what you were wearing the last time you arrived home. How does that memory differ from remembering which months of the year have 30 days in them, or naming the prime numbers between 20 and 30, or remembering how to make an omelette? These might feel like different kinds of memory, in intuitive terms. But what is the scientific evidence? In fact, one of the major findings over the past 100 years is that memory is a multicomponent (rather than monolithic) entity. We discuss these distinctions further in this chapter, and elsewhere in this book.

In the 1960s, subdivisions of memory based upon information-processing models became popular. Following rapid developments in information technology that took place after the Second World War, there was substantial growth in understanding the requirements of information storage during computer processing. A three-stage model of memory processing subsequently developed, reaching its fullest elaboration in the model proposed by Atkinson and Shiffrin in the 1960s. In these stage models, information was considered to be first held very briefly in *sensory memories*, after which a selection of this information was transferred to a *short-term store*. From here, a yet smaller amount of information made its way into a *long-term memory store*.

MULTI-STORE MODEL

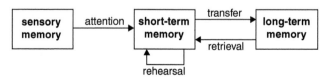

5. Multistore (or modal) model of memory, first described in 1968 by Atkinson and Shiffrin. This model has offered a very useful heuristic framework for an understanding of memory

The characteristics of these different stores are outlined below.

Sensory store

The sensory store (Figure 5) appears to operate below the threshold of consciousness. It receives information from the senses and holds it for about a second while we decide what to attend to. An example of this is the 'cocktail party phenomenon', where – in the middle of another conversation – we may hear our name mentioned in a conversation elsewhere in the room, which then automatically diverts our attention to that other conversation. Another common experience is that we may ask someone to repeat an action or re-state something that they said (believing it has been forgotten), while at the same time we discover that we do, in fact, have access to the information with which we have been previously presented. With sensory memory, what we ignore is quickly lost and cannot be retrieved: it decays just as – from a sensory perspective – lights fade and sounds die away. So you can sometimes catch an echo of what someone said when you are not paying attention, but a second later it has gone altogether.

Objective evidence for *sensory memory* stores came from experiments such as that conducted by Sperling in 1960. Sperling presented displays of 12 letters very briefly (e.g. for 50 milliseconds) to participants. Although participants in this study could report only about four letters, Sperling suspected that the participants might actually be able to remember more letters, but the information faded too rapidly for it to be reported. In order to test this hypothesis, Sperling very cleverly designed a visual matrix, in which the letters were presented in three rows. Very shortly after the presentation of the visual array, a tone was sounded. Participants were instructed to report only part of the visual array, according to the pitch of the tone. Using this *partial report procedure*, Sperling found that people could recall about three letters from any row of four letters – indicating that, for just a very brief period, about nine out of the twelve letters were potentially reportable.

Memory researchers inferred from research such as this that a sensory memory store exists, holding a relatively large amount of incoming perceptual information very briefly while selected elements are processed. The sensory memory for visual information has been termed *iconic memory*, while sensory memory for auditory information has been referred to as *echoic memory*. Sensory memories are generally characterized as being rich (in terms of their content) but very brief (in terms of their duration).

Short-term memory

Beyond the sensory memories, information-processing models advocated in the 1960s hypothesized one or more short-term stores that held information for a few seconds (Figure 5). Paying attention to something transfers it to short-term memory (sometimes referred to as *primary memory* or the *short-term store*), which has a capacity of around seven items. This store is used when, for example, dialling a new phone number. It has limited capacity, so that – once short-term memory is full – old information is displaced by new input. Less important thoughts (e.g. a phone number you have to call today but will never need again) are held in short-term memory, used, and then decay. For example, if you're going to phone the cinema to find out what films are showing this evening, you need to hold the phone number in mind for a relatively short period and then it can be discarded.

Within the scientific literature, the verbal short-term store has received considerable attention. Its existence has been inferred – at least in part – from the *recency effect* in free recall. For example, Postman and Phillips asked their participants to recall lists of 10, 20 or 30 words. On immediate recall, the participants tended to be much better at recalling the last few words that had been presented than they were at recalling words from the middle of the list, known as the recency effect. But this effect disappeared if memory testing was delayed by as little as 15 seconds (as long as the delay involved verbal activity by the participant, such as counting backwards). The interpretation of these findings was that the recency effect involved the last few memory items being retrieved from a short-term store of rather limited capacity.

It was further suggested by Alan Baddeley in the 1960s that the verbal short-term store retained information primarily in an acoustic or phonological form. This view received support from noting the acoustic nature of the errors that appear during short-term recall. This occurred even when the material to be retained was presented visually, indicating that the stored information was converted to an acoustic code. For example, Conrad and Hull showed that visually presented sequences of letters that are similar in sound (e.g. P, D, B, V, C, T) were harder to recall correctly after presentation than were sequences of dissimilar-sounding letters (e.g. W, K, L, Y, R, Z).

Long-term memory

Continuing to attend to and turn over in one's mind (or 'rehearse') information transfers it to the long-term store (sometimes referred to as *secondary memory*), which seems to have almost unlimited capacity. More important information (for example, the new phone number that you have to learn when you move house, your bank PIN, or your date of birth) is placed in the long term store (Figure 5). It is this long-term aspect of memory that is the primary focus of this chapter.

By contrast with acoustic representation of information in the short-term store, information in long-term memory is thought to be stored primarily in terms of the *meaning* of the information. So, when asked to remember later on a selection of meaningful sentences which were presented earlier, people usually cannot reproduce the exact wording, but they can generally report the meaning or gist of the sentences. As we saw in Chapter 1 (when considering the work of Bartlett) the 'top down' imposing of meaning can often lead to distortions and biases in memory, as in the case of the *The War of the Ghosts* story. We will return to this topic of bias in long-term memory in Chapter 4, when we consider *eyewitness testimony*.

Models like Atkinson and Shiffrin's three stage model of memory, outlined above, are useful for simplifying and representing some aspects of the complexity of human memory (Figure 5). However, this very complexity requires ongoing adjustment to enable these models to incorporate additional observations. For example, the information-processing model outlined above made two fundamental assumptions: i. information could only reach long-term memory by first passing through the short-term store; and ii. rehearsing information in the short-term store would both retain it in this store, and increase its chance of being transferred to the long-term store.

However, the first of these assumptions was challenged by the identification of key clinical cases. These brain-injured patients manifested grossly impaired short-term memory capacity and therefore (in terms of the Atkinson-Shiffrin model) severely damaged short-term memory stores. However, these patients appeared to have no impairment in their long-term memory ability. The second assumption of the Atkinson-Shiffrin model was challenged by the findings of studies in which participants rehearsed the last few words of word lists for a longer time period, without showing improvement in the long-term recall of those words. Under some circumstances, it also became clear that encountering the same information on many different occasions (which may, reasonably, be assumed to lead to increased rehearsal) was not sufficient to lead to the retention of this information. For example, as we saw in Chapter 1, people do not perform very well when they are asked to remember the details on the faces of the coins that they handle on a daily basis.

Other evidence for the distinction between short-term and long-term memory stores has also come into question. For example, as we saw previously, the recency effect in free recall had been attributed to the operation of a short-term store, because this effect was reduced when the few seconds before recall were filled with a verbal task such as backward counting. But when participants studied words and counted backwards after each word in the list, the last few items were still better recalled than the middle of the list. This pattern of findings was at odds with the Atkinson and Shiffrin model, because the short-term store should have been 'filled' with the backwards counting task – and so no recency effect should have been observed. Semantic encoding (that is, processing information in terms of its meaning) has also been demonstrated in short-term learning under suitable conditions, indicating that phonological encoding is not the only form of coding relevant for the representation of information in the short-term store.

Two major responses followed recognition of the problems with Atkinson and Shiffrin's information-processing model (Figure 5). One approach, especially associated with Baddeley and colleagues, was to refine the short-term memory model in the light of its known limitations. Baddeley and colleagues also sought to characterize further the functions that short-term remembering plays in cognition. This change in perspective led to Baddeley's original – and subsequently revised – working memory model. The other main response to the problems identified with Atkinson and Shiffrin's model was – more generally – to question the emphasis placed in this model on memory stores and their capacity limitations, and to focus instead on an alternative approach based on the nature of the processing that takes place in memory, and the consequences of this processing for remembering.

Whichever specific memory model is ultimately the most compelling, many theories of memory make a general but fundamental distinction between short-term and long-term memory processes. As we will see, evidence for a dichotomy between the short-term and long-term memory store comes from i) a range of experiments that have been conducted on healthy individuals, and ii) the study of brain-injured patients with deficits in memory. There is also convergent evidence from fundamental biological research supporting the distinction between short- and long-term memory storage.

Working memory

Considering further the short-term store, the distinction between *short-term memory* and *working memory* is often blurred. Short-term memory was previously conceptualized (either explicitly or implicitly) as a relatively *passive* process. But we now know that people do more than just hold information in the short-term store. For example, if we have a sentence held in our short-term memory, we can usually repeat the words in the sentence in reverse order, or recite the first letter of each word in the sentence. It is this more *active* sense of short-term memory that is denoted by the use of the term working memory, because there are some mental operations (or 'work') being done on the information that is currently held in mind. The terms 'working memory' and 'short-term memory' are also often used synonymously with *consciousness*. This is because what we're consciously aware of – that is, what we're currently holding in mind – is held within our working memory.

The term *span* is often used to refer to the amount of information that a person is able to hold within short-term memory. For healthy young people, George Miller in the 1950s defined the limits of short-term memory as typically 7 ± 2 items. The mechanisms underpinning our short-term memory can be demonstrated when we try to remember a list of words: we tend to remember the last few words in the list best, because these words are still held within our short-term memory. As noted by William Shakespeare in *Richard II* 'As the last taste of sweets, is sweetest last, writ in remembrance more than things long past.' It has been suggested that short-term memory span is linked with speech articulation speed, so the faster somebody can say words or letters or numbers under their breath, the longer their short-term memory span.

There's now good evidence that working memory is not a single entity, but that it is made up of at least three components (see Figure 6). Baddeley has formalized these components in his influential working memory model as a *central executive* and two so-called 'slave' systems – the *phonological loop* and the *visuo-spatial sketchpad*. Subsequently, Baddeley added an *episodic buffer* in his revised working memory model. With respect to the proposed functional roles of these components, it is proposed that i) the central executive controls attention and coordinates the slave systems, ii) the phonological loop contains a phonological store and an articulatory control process and is responsible for inner speech, iii) the visuo-spatial sketchpad is responsible for setting up and manipulating mental images, and iv) the episodic buffer (not shown) integrates and manipulates material in working memory.

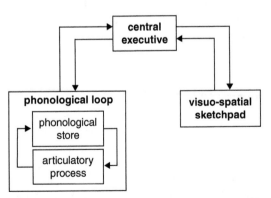

6. In 1974, Alan Baddeley and Graham Hitch proposed a working memory model which subdivided short-term memory into three basic components: the central executive, the phonological loop and the visuo-spatial sketchpad

Phonological loop

A considerable amount of research has been concentrated on the *phonological* (or *articulatory*) *loop*. It is thought to play an important role in language development, and in comprehension of complex linguistic materials in adults. Its existence is supported by experiments showing that performance on memory span tasks typically depends substantially on the use of an articulatory code. For example, the number of words that you can hear and then repeat back without error is a function of the complexity of the words. By using a technique known as *articulatory suppression*, in which research participants repeat (aloud or silently) a simple sound or word, such as 'la la la' or 'the the the', the phonological loop can be prevented temporarily from retaining any further information. So contrasting performance with and without articulatory suppression can be used to demonstrate the contribution of the phonological loop.

The phonological loop has a finite length. Is this length best characterized in terms of a number of items or a period of time? It has been shown that one's *memory span* – i.e. the number of words that one can hear and then repeat back without error – is a function of the length of time that it takes to say the words. So, a word list like 'cold, cat, France, Kansas, iron' is considerably easier to remember on a short-term memory test than 'emphysema, rhinoceros, Mozambique, Connecticut, magnesium', even though the two lists are matched in terms of the number of words and the semantic categories from which they are drawn (namely: diseases, animals, countries, American states and metals). However, this *word length effect* is eliminated if participants have to carry out articulatory suppression while they study the word list. Another example of the word length effects comes from the varying speed with which the digits 1-10 can be pronounced in different languages: the size of the digit memory span for people who speak different languages is highly correlated with the speed with which the digits can be spoken in that language. These and other findings indicate that the phonological loop is time- (rather than item-) limited.

Visuo-spatial sketchpad

By contrast, the *visuo-spatial sketchpad* provides a medium for the temporary storage and manipulation of images. Its existence is inferred from studies showing that concurrent spatial tasks interfere with each other with respect to short-term memory capacity. So, if you try to perform two non-verbal tasks simultaneously (for example, patting your head and rubbing your tummy), these two tasks combined may be overworking the visuo-spatial sketchpad, and so performance on each task declines (relative to the level of performance when each task is performed alone). Studies have indicated that the visuo-spatial sketchpad is involved in playing chess – reflecting the contribution of spatial short-term memory in processing the different configurations of chess pieces on a board.

Central executive

This is, to date, the least well characterized component of Baddeley's working memory model. It is thought to mediate the attentional and strategic aspects of working memory, and may be involved in co-ordinating cognitive resources between the phonological loop and the visuo-spatial sketchpad, if both are active simultaneously – for example, if you are trying to remember a word list and perform a spatial movement at the same time (as we have asked participants to do in some of our own research). In studying the central executive, Baddeley and colleagues have applied such a dual task methodology, in which one of the tasks (the first task) is designed to keep the central executive busy, while the second task is evaluated for whether the central executive is involved in the performance of this task. When performance on the second task suffers due to the concurrent performance of the first task, it can be concluded that the central executive is involved in performing the second task. One task used by researchers to engage the central executive is the generation of random letter sequences. Participants are required to generate letter sequences, taking care to avoid sequences of letters that fall into meaningful orders, such as 'C-A-T', 'A-B-C', or 'S-U-V'. Participants' generation and monitoring of their letter choices occupies the central executive. It has been shown that the memory of expert chess players for positions taken from actual chess games was impaired by performance of the letter generation task but not by articulatory suppression, indicating that the central executive (but not the phonological loop) was involved in remembering the chess positions. From a clinical perspective, the effects of disruption of the central executive can be seen in the kind of disorganized and unplanned behaviour observed in the 'dysexecutive syndrome' (which has been linked to frontal lobe brain damage; see Chapters 5 and 6).

The episodic buffer

The most recent version of Baddeley's working memory model introduced this functional component. According to Baddeley's revised model, information that is retrieved from long-term memory often needs to be integrated with respect to the current demands being fulfilled by working memory. Baddeley (2001) attributes this cognitive function to the episodic buffer. Baddeley provides the example of our being able to imagine an elephant playing ice-hockey. Within this framework, it is argued that we can go beyond the information about elephants and ice-hockey supplied to us from long-term memory by imagining that the elephant is pink, by picturing how the elephant holds the hockey stick, and by reflecting on what field position the elephant might occupy. So, the episodic buffer allows us to extrapolate beyond what already exists in long-term memory, to combine it in different ways, and to use it to create novel scenarios on which future actions can be based.

Memory metaphors

Working memory could be likened to the RAM capacity of your desktop computer. The operations that are currently being engaged in by the computer – in terms of its processing resources – are occupying RAM, the computer's 'working memory'. The hard disk of the computer is like long-term memory, so you can put information onto the hard disk and store it there indefinitely, and it's still stored there when you switch off the computer overnight. Switching off power to the computer might be regarded as analogous to falling asleep for humans! After a good night's sleep, we still have access to information stored in our long-term memory (such as our name, our date of birth, how many siblings we have, and what happened on an especially eventful day in our personal past) when we wake up the next morning. But, typically, we cannot remember the last thoughts that we were holding in our working memory when we wake up the next morning (because this information was usually not transferred into our long-term memory before we fell asleep – this can be very frustrating for those of us who generate our best ideas in the few minutes before we enter the land of Nod!). Another relevant comparison concerns i) the use of short-term memory in making a one-off phone call to a restaurant that one has never visited before, versus ii) the creation of new long-term memories when, for example, we move to a new house and may have to create a memory representation of our new home phone number.

The computer disk drive analogy also helps us to understand the distinction between encoding, storage, and retrieval in memory. Think about the huge amount of information on the Internet. This can be thought of as a massive long-term memory system. But, without effective tools for searching and retrieving information from the Internet, that information is essentially useless: it may be theoretically available, but is it practically accessible when you need it? This is why the advent of effective search tools such as

Google and Yahoo have massively transformed the use of the Internet in recent years.

Moving beyond working memory and its proposed component processes, we now consider the different functional elements that have been proposed within long-term memory. These distinctions have been proposed as a means of characterizing the findings that have been obtained in the memory literature through the evaluation of both healthy individuals and people with different forms of brain injury. Both of these sources have provided valuable information pertaining to the organization of human memory.

Semantic, episodic, and procedural memory

One potentially useful distinction made by psychologists is between *episodic memory* and *semantic memory*, each of which is considered to represent a different type of consciously accessible long-term memory (this distinction was already mentioned in Chapter 1). In particular, Tulving has argued that *episodic memory* involves remembering specific events, whereas *semantic memory* essentially concerns general knowledge about the world. Episodic memory includes recollection of *time*, *place*, and associated *emotions* at the time of the event. (*Autobiographical memory* – the recall of events from our earlier life – represents a sub-category of episodic memory that has attracted considerable interest in recent years).

Put concisely, episodic memory can be defined as memory for the events of your life that you have experienced. These memories naturally tend to retain details of the time and situation in which they were acquired. So remembering what you did last weekend, or recollecting what happened when you took your driving test, would comprise examples of episodic memory.

Episodic memory contrasts and interacts with *semantic memory*, the memory of *facts* and *concepts*. *Semantic memory* can be defined as knowledge that is retained irrespective of the circumstances under which it was acquired. In fact, we often combine and conflate episodic and semantic memory without being aware that we are doing so; for example, when trying to recall what happened on our wedding day, our actual recollections of the day may well be combined with our expectations and semantic knowledge abut the kinds of things that typically happen at weddings.

Here are some examples to illustrate *semantic memory*:

What is the capital of France?
How many days are there in the week?
Who is the current Prime Minister of the United Kingdom?
Tell me the name of a mammal that flies.
What is the chemical symbol for water?
What direction would you travel in if you were flying from London to Johannesburg?

These are questions with relative degrees of difficulty, but all of them tap into the huge store of general knowledge about the world that we acquire throughout our lives and which we tend to take for granted. In contrast, if I asked you what you had for breakfast yesterday, or what happened on your last birthday, your response would draw on your *episodic memory*, because I'm now asking you questions about specific events, or episodes, that have occurred in your life. So, your memory of eating breakfast this morning will be an episodic memory involving when, where, and what you ate. On the other hand, remembering what the term 'breakfast' means and refers to involves semantic memory. So, you can no doubt describe what 'breakfast' means, but you probably have no recollection of when and how you learned the concept – unless you learned abut the concept of breakfast very recently (you no doubt learned about 'breakfast' as a child, but there may well be other concepts that you have acquired much more recently). How episodic memories become 'converted' into semantic memories over time remains an area of considerable research interest and speculation (for example, the first time you leaned about Mt Everest being the world's tallest mountain was within a specific episode, but gradually over time – and repeated exposure – this information became converted into a piece of semantic information).

Whether semantic and episodic memory represent truly separate memory systems is still quite uncertain. But the distinction has been quite useful in helping to characterize clinical memory disorders which appear to affect one system more than the other. For example, researchers have found that there are certain disorders of the brain that can preferentially affect semantic memory, such as 'semantic dementia'. In contrast, Endel Tulving has argued that the so-called 'amnesic syndrome' is characterized by a selective impairment in episodic memory, but not in semantic memory (see Chapter 5).

There seems to be general agreement that a third type of long-term memory – *procedural memory* (for example, performing the sequence of physical operations necessary to be able to ride a bicycle) – is independent of consciously accessible memory. Again, there appear to be certain disorders of the brain that can preferentially affect procedural memory, such as Parkinson's disease. There have also been suggestions that procedural memory should not be considered as a homogenous memory system, but that – instead – procedural memory comprises several different subsystems.

Explicit and implicit memory

Another common distinction made by memory researchers is that between explicit and implicit memory. (This proposed framework bears some similarities to the framework discussed in the last section – involving episodic, semantic, and procedural memory.) Within this framework, e*xplicit memory* is defined as involving conscious awareness, at the time of remembering, of the information, experience, or situation being remembered. Other researchers have referred to this type of memory experience as 'recollective', rather than explicit. There are close parallels here with episodic memory, previously discussed.

Implicit memory, by contrast, refers to an influence on behaviour, feelings or thoughts as a result of prior experience, but which is manifested without conscious recollection of the original events. For example, if you pass a Chinese restaurant on the way to work in the morning, you might later that day think about going out for a Chinese meal, without being consciously aware that this disposition had been influenced by the experience that you had that morning.

Distinctions between implicit and explicit memory are sometimes demonstrated by studies that measure a phenomenon termed 'priming'. One task used in many priming studies is timed completion of word fragments (such as e_e_h_n_; turn to page 48 to see if you completed this fragment correctly). In healthy individuals, completions of fragmented words are generally faster or more certain for recently encountered words than for new ones. Odd as it may seem, this phenomenon occurs even when the words are not themselves consciously remembered but can still access implicit memory. A complementary source of evidence for the implicit/explicit distinction again comes from studies involving patients with *amnesia*. In these patients, their amnesia means that they cannot consciously recognize words or pictures that have been previously presented to them, but – like healthy individuals – they are nevertheless better at completing the corresponding word fragments later on. These studies suggest that there is a fundamental difference in the functional characteristics of memory, depending upon whether the test requires conscious awareness of the previous event.

There is further evidence for this view. For example, in the 1980s Larry Jacoby conducted a study in which there were two types of test: 'recognition' (involving conscious remembering of the studied information) and 'unconscious remembering' (in this case, this was tested via a perceptual identification task, i.e. identifying a visually presented word that appeared very briefly). Jacoby also manipulated how the target words were studied in this experiment. Each target word was shown either a) with no context (e.g. 'girl' shown alone), or b) shown with its opposite as a context (e.g. 'boy – girl' shown together), or c) generated by the participant when shown its opposite (e.g. 'boy' was shown and 'girl' was generated by the participant).

The subsequent explicit memory test involved showing a mixture of target words and new words to participants, and asking them to identify which words they had studied previously ('studied' words included both read and generated words, as described in the previous paragraph). By contrast, for the implicit memory test a mixture of targets and new words were shown very briefly, one at a time, and the participants were asked to identify each word as it was presented. The findings of this study were as follows: explicit recognition improved from the 'no context' condition to the 'generate' condition, but – interestingly – the reverse was the case for the implicit perceptual identification task! Because the pattern of results was reversed for the two tests, it suggests that the underlying processes (i.e. implicit and explicit memories) are distinct, and involve possibly independent memory mechanisms.

The study described in the last paragraph represents a good example of how carefully defined experimentation can help us to establish a key difference between mental processes that we would be unable to separate reliably using self-reflection or introspection. Another example of careful, systematic research in this field concerns the work of Andrade and others into memory during general anaesthesia. These researchers have demonstrated that people can subsequently show implicit memory for materials presented to them during anaesthesia, even when they are unconscious at the time of presentation. Findings such as this have led to suggestions that members of surgical teams should be especially careful what they say about patients during an operation conducted under general anaesthetic! In addition, further research has suggested that commercial advertising may work primarily through its effects on implicit memory. It has been demonstrated that when people who have been shown adverts previously are asked to rate these adverts again later, they rate the previously seen adverts as being more attractive than adverts that they have not seen previously (a phenomenon known as the *mere exposure effect*).

Different kinds of memory task

The implicit/explicit memory distinction represents a distinction regarding two proposed memory systems (see Foster and Jelicic, 1999, for a more technical, comprehensive review of this topic). This distinction between two proposed memory systems is often used – and potentially confused with – different types of *memory task*, in which different functional processes may be differentially involved. Some memory tasks require people to think about meanings and concepts; these are often referred to as *concept-driven tasks*. For example, if you are asked to remember items from a list of words that you studied, then you would be explicitly recalling the words themselves. At the same time, you would be likely to recall automatically the meanings of the words too. Other tasks require people to focus more on the perceptual aspects of the presented materials; these are often referred to as *data-driven tasks*. So if your task was to complete word fragments (such as e_e_h_n_) without reference to the studied list, then the influence of the study session would likely be more implicit rather than explicit; you would be working with the visual patterns of letters, but less so (if at all) with the word meanings.

Tasks that are proposed to tap, differentially, into explicit and implicit memory are sometimes also called *direct* and *indirect* memory tasks, respectively. It is challenging to separate the nature of the task (i.e. concept- or data-driven; direct versus indirect) and the nature of the memory component being tested (i.e. explicit or implicit). Indeed, many researchers have argued that no memory task is truly 'process pure', in that each memory task will be mediated by a combination of implicit and explicit processes – it is the weighting of these processes that will differ across different memory tasks.

The experience of memory

Related to the explicit/implicit memory distinction is the type of remembering experience that accompanies performance on a memory task. For example, it has been proposed that there is a valid distinction in memory between a person 'remembering' and 'knowing' something. 'Remembering' has been defined in terms of someone having a phenomenological experience that they saw the specific item under test on the original learning trial. By contrast, it has been suggested that a person may simply 'know' that the word was in the original list, without that person specifically recalling the item. This 'remember'/'know' distinction was first used by Endel Tulving. In his research, Tulving required each response at test to be judged as being either a) an experience of remembering having studied the item, or b) knowing that the item had been presented, but without specifically remembering the event. Gardiner, Java, and colleagues have since carried out a range investigations of 'remember/know' judgements under a variety of different experimental conditions.

This distinction may be somewhat difficult to operationalize, that is to characterize in objective terms. However, a number of experimental manipulations have been shown to influence 'remember' and 'know' judgements differently. For example, studies have shown that semantic processing (where the meaning of the items is emphasized) leads to more 'remember' responses than does acoustic processing (which focuses on the sound of the words studied). In contrast, research findings indicate that the proportion of 'know' responses does not differ between semantic and acoustic conditions.

Levels of processing

One complementary framework that has been very influential when thinking about memory (especially long-term memory) is the 'levels of processing' framework. In contrast to structural models of memory, this framework emphasizes the importance of processing in memory, rather than structure and capacity. The levels of framework approach was first articulated in the experimental psychology literature by Fergus Craik and Bob Lockhart, but its key principle was in some senses foreshadowed anecdotally by the novelist Marcel Proust when he wrote: 'We soon forget what we have not deeply thought about'. Craik and Lockhart argued that how well we remember depends on how well we process information at the time of encoding. They described different *levels of processing*, from 'superficial' levels that deal only with the physical properties of the presented stimuli, through 'deeper' processes involving phonological properties, down to yet deeper processes that involve semantic encoding of the material in terms of its meaning.

Subsequently, many formal experiments have shown that – in terms of later memory performance at test – 'deeper' processing of information at encoding is superior to more 'superficial' processing, and that elaboration of material via semantic processing can improve learning of memory materials. What does this mean? Well, here is an example. Suppose you were asked to study a list of words and a) provide a definition of each word on the list, or b) provide a personal association for each word on the list (both of which require semantic processing of the words on the list). You would typically remember the list of words better under conditions a) or b) than if you were asked to perform a more superficial and less semantic task, such as c) providing another rhyming word for each word on the list, or d) providing a letter number from the alphabet corresponding to each letter in each word on the list.

In other words, if we see the word 'DOG', we might simply process it in a relatively superficial manner by noting that it is written in upper case. On the other hand, we might process it phonologically by registering that its sound rhymes with 'frog' and 'log'. Alternatively, we could think about the meaning of the word: 'dog' refers to domesticated, hairy animals sometimes referred to as 'man's best friend'. Further semantic processing, involving elaboration based on the meaning of the word, represents deeper processing, and should lead to better memory (for example, we might think about different breeds of dog, where they originate, their original functional roles, the characteristics of the breed, and so on).

Demonstrating the usefulness of this approach, Craik and Tulving showed that the probability of the same word being correctly recognized in a memory experiment varied from 20% to 70%, depending on the 'depth' of processing that had been previously carried out at the time of encoding. When the initial processing involved only decisions about the letter case in which the word was printed, correct recognition occurred at the 20% level. Performance improved following rhyming (i.e. phonological) decisions, but was considerably better (i.e. almost 70% correct recognition) when processing involved decisions about whether the word would fit meaningfully into a given sentence.

A considerable volume of data supports the levels of processing model. However, the details of the original model have been criticized. Specifically, objections have been raised on the grounds that this approach is logically circular in its mode of explanation. So, if it is observed that a particular encoding operation or procedure produces better memory performance, then it can be argued – in terms of the 'levels of processing' framework – that this arises from a 'deeper' mode of cognitive processing. If, by contrast, another encoding operation or procedure produced poorer subsequent memory performance, then – according to the 'level of processing' account – this must have been due to more 'superficial' processing at the time of encoding. So the central concern is that the 'levels of processing' framework thereby becomes self-fulfilling and untestable. The problem – in essence – is how to devise a criterion of 'depth' and 'shallowness' of processing that is independent of subsequent memory performance.

It has therefore been argued that a level of processing criterion cannot be identified independently of the memory performance that it produces. More recently, however, Fergus Craik has pointed to physiological and neurological methods that may provide an independent measure of depth of processing. Notwithstanding possible problems with the testability of the model, a 'levels of processing' approach does – importantly – draw attention to important functional issues including a) the type of processing of materials at the time of encoding, b) elaboration of materials during encoding, and c) the appropriateness of the processing that takes place at the time of encoding (in terms of 'transfer' to the later memory task; this issue will be considered further in Chapter 3). Similar to the framework articulated by Bartlett (Chapter 1), a key emphasis from the levels of processing framework is that we are *active agents* in the remembering process, such that what we remember depends on i) the processes that we ourselves engage in when we encounter a thing or an event, as well as ii) the properties of the thing or event itself.

Word fragment (from page 42)

Elephant

Chapter 3
Pulling the rabbit out of the hat

If you want to test your memory, try to recall what you were worrying about one year ago today.

Anonymous

This chapter will consider how information is accessed from memory. I will consider the key distinction between information accessibility and availability, already alluded to in Chapter 2. In particular, I will make the point that many of the everyday difficulties that we experience with our memory relate to situations in which we may have taken in and retained the information, but we are unable to retrieve that information when we wish to do so. The role of context seems to be especially important here: other things being equal, we tend to remember information better if we are in a similar physical context and emotional state at the time we wish to retrieve information as we were in at the time we were exposed to that information. The 'tip of the tongue phenomenon' will also be examined further in this chapter. For example, at a party we may know the first letter of a name (of a person or place) that we are trying to recall, or what the name sounds like, but we may not be able to access the name itself.

Inferring memory from behaviour

As we saw in Chapter 2, there are many sorts of behaviour that suggest that a memory has been evoked for some past event.

Suppose you heard a new song some time ago. Later, you might recall the words of the song, or recognize the words when you hear them again. Alternatively, if you hear the song again, the words might sound familiar without your explicitly recognizing them. Finally, your behaviour or mental state might be covertly influenced by the message of the song, without your having any sense of conscious recall, recognition or familiarity for the song itself.

Every day we encounter an enormous quantity of information, but we only remember some of it. Having encoded and stored information that has been processed by our senses, we then have to be able to retrieve it effectively – as we saw when considering the fundamental logical components of memory in Chapter 1. Which events we remember seems to depend on their functional significance. For example, in our evolutionary past, humans may have survived by remembering information that signalled threat (such as the appearance of a potential predator) or reward (such as the discovery of a possible food source).

What we are able to retrieve depends largely on the context in which the information was encoded or classified in the first place, and to what extent this matches the retrieval context – this is the so-called *encoding specificity principle* (as articulated by Endel Tulving). For example, many of us have been somewhat embarrassed by our inability to recognize friends or acquaintances when we meet them in an unusual context. If we habitually see someone at work or school dressed in a particular way, we may fail to recognize them if we see them dressed very differently at a wedding or in a restaurant. We consider this principle further below. But first we consider a few key methods for assessing memory.

Retrieval: recall versus recognition

To *recall* information is to bring it to mind. Usually there is some *cue* that triggers and/or facilitates the recall. For example, examination questions typically contain content cues that direct our recall to information relevant to the examiner's aims. Everyday questions such as 'What did you do on Friday night?' contain time cues. Cues such as these are very general, and do not provide a great deal of information. Recall in response to these sorts of non-specific cues is generally termed *free recall*. Some cues may also be more informative and direct us to more specific events or information. A question such as 'Where did you go on Friday night after you left the movies?' differs from the previous question, cited above, by providing us with more information in an effort to extract some specific material. As cues become more directive, the recall process is termed *cued recall.*

Here are some other examples. When investigating retrieval in an experimental context, people might be presented with information, such as a story, during what we call the learning episode. Then we may ask them to recall certain aspects of the story. *Free recall* is where we ask people to remember as much of the story as they can, without any assistance. The 'tip of the tongue phenomenon' (mentioned in Chapter 2) illustrates the nature of one common problem in free recall, in that we often have only partial access to information that we're trying to retrieve. By comparison, *cued recall* is where we present a prompt (such as a category, or the first letter of the word) in order to retrieve a certain piece of information. For example, we might say 'Tell me all the names of people beginning with 'J' that were in the story that I read to you yesterday'. Cued recall tends to be somewhat easier for respondents than free recall. This may be because we're providing more support and context for the individual – i.e. we are actually doing some of the 'memory work' for them in providing these cues. It should be noted that cues can be useful in retrieving information, but they can also introduce distortion and bias – as we will see in more detail when we consider the issue of eyewitness testimony in Chapter 4.

Our ability to identify some past event or information when it is presented to us again is termed *recognition*. For example, in examinations, true–false and multiple-choice questions typically target the student's ability to recognize information correctly. In real life, questions like 'Did you go out to eat after you left the movies?' present some event or information and ask the person concerned whether it matches the past. *Recognition* is the easiest type of retrieval, because some of the 'target' memory material is actually presented, and you – the respondent – have to make a decision about it. 'Forced choice recognition' is where you are presented with, say, two items – only one of which you've seen previously – and you are asked 'Tell me which of these two items you saw before'. It's a forced choice, in that you have to choose one of the two items. This can be compared with 'yes/no recognition', where I would show you a series of items one at a time and ask 'Did you see this item before?'. In this case, you simply have to answer 'yes' or 'no' in response to each item. Systematic experiments have indicated that two independent processes can contribute to recognition:

Context retrieval

This depends on 'explicit recollection' of time and place; for example, you may recognize someone as the person you saw on the bus when you were coming home from work last Friday. So for this type of recognition, you need to be able to locate your previous experience in time and place.

Familiarity

You may see someone who looks vaguely familiar, and you know you've seen them before, but you can't quite remember when or where you saw them. This type of recognition experience seems to be served by a 'familiarity process', but there is no explicit recollection of the previous encounter. This is, therefore, a less detailed form of recognition (very similar to the 'know' type of response that we discussed in Chapter 2). Effects on familiarity can be noted without the ability to bring to mind (that is, recall or recognize) a past event. You have probably had this experience yourself on several occasions: i.e. you have encountered someone

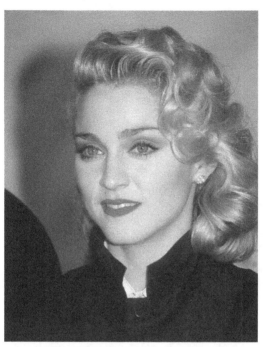

7. You may well be able to recall the identity of this person spontaneously, or you may require a cue (such as 'singer' or 'entertainer'). If you cannot recall the name of this person, you may be able to recognize her name: is it Cher or Madonna? Cued recall tends to be somewhat easier for respondents than free recall, while recognition tends to be easier than either free or cued recall

who seemed familiar, although you were unable to recognize them explicitly. Indeed, one of the mechanisms underlying the success of advertising is that it makes particular products more familiar, and people tend to prefer familiar things to more unfamiliar ones. (Please refer to the *mere exposure effect* cited in Chapter 2). Hence the old adage, 'All publicity is good publicity.'

There is a curious phenomenon that most of us have experienced which may be centrally dependent on the feeling of misplaced familiarity: déjà vu. This phenomenon occurs when people feel they have witnessed something before, without being quite able to place the prior event or provide any further confirmatory evidence that the event or incident actually took place. It seems that in déjà vu, familiarity mechanisms may occur by mistake, so that a feeling of familiarity is triggered by a novel object or scene. Furthermore, it has been suggested by some researchers that déjà vu can be induced by hypnosis. So it seems possible that the brain mechanisms underlying the experience of déjà vu may be mediated by different mechanisms than those that typically operate when we are fully alert.

The effect of context on recall and recognition

Recall can be quite susceptible to the effects of context, but recognition is typically less susceptible. This has been shown, for example, in divers who were asked to remember information underwater or on dry land, and then had their memory tested either in the same location or in a different location.

In two famous studies, Godden and Baddeley asked divers to remember information either on the shore or underwater. The divers were then tested either a) in the same context, or b) in a different context.

These studies showed that the divers' recall memory was strongly influenced by whether they were in the same context when they encoded the information as they were in for the memory test. So the divers remembered far more information if they were asked to learn underwater and then were tested underwater, or if they learned on land and then were tested on land. But if the context in which they learned and were tested was different – underwater to land, or land to underwater – then the divers' level of memory performance dropped markedly. In summary, the divers experienced difficulties with recall when they had to remember information in a different location, but not when they remembered information in the same location as during learning.

However, this was only evident for recall, not for recognition memory. So it seems as if the cues that are provided by being in the same context at learning and test are important in effective recall, but less influential for recognition.

Interestingly, recall performance is also influenced by a person's physiological or psychological state. For example, if someone learns something while they're very calm and then is tested when they're very anxious or excited, then their recall performance level tends to be impaired. But if they learn while calm and then are memory tested while calm, or learn while they are excited and then are tested while excited, then their performance tends to be better. This is significant for students studying for exams: if you revise for an exam while you are very calm, but then feel very nervous or excited in the actual examination, then you might not recall information so well in the examination (compared with someone whose mood is more even across study and test). So relaxation therapy may be advisable for you in such circumstances, to try to ensure that you are in a similar psychological and physiological state at the time of the exam as you were when you were revising.

Alcohol and other agents and drugs which influence one's psychological state have been noted to have similar effects. In subjective terms, this point was captured quite well by the comedian and entertainer Billy Connolly, when he was interviewed on Australian television in 2006:

> Oh I remember now where I was, oh yeah I remember doing that and I remember doing this and then you go to the next stage which is black outs that you don't remember, so in order to remember them you have to get drunk again so you get two memories. You've got a sober memory and a drunk memory because you've become two guys . . .

(ABC transcript of *Enough Rope* interview)

So we observe these *state-dependent* memory and forgetting effects, as well as physical *context-dependent* effects.

State-dependent effects on memory seem to occur under a variety of different circumstances, but – in systematic experimental studies – they are also found consistently only when memory is tested using free recall. When either cued recall or recognition is tested, the influence of changes in state or context is quite variable.

Although the question is difficult to study scientifically, it is likely that one of the reasons we find it challenging to recall the contents of dreams is related to state-dependent forgetting. However, if we are awakened while we are actually dreaming, we typically find it relatively straightforward to recall some of the dream – probably because at least some of the content of the dream is still held in working memory.

Several factors may explain the state-dependent sensitivity of free recall. For example, different psycho-active states could lead people to adopt unusual encoding or retrieval strategies which are incompatible which those they use when they are not in those states. Marijuana intoxication, for instance, causes people to make unusual associations in reaction to stimuli. This could be critical in mediating free recall, because here the participant has to generate appropriate contextual cues or information to aid their remembering. But in cued recall and recognition, some information is actually provided about the target items to the respondent, and so the potential for a mismatch between encoding and retrieval operations is substantially reduced – because a certain amount of the information that had been presented at the time of learning is re-presented at the time of test (and is therefore constant).

In addition – as we saw earlier – recognition memory often has a strong 'familiarity' component, which is context-free, and therefore not vulnerable to context shifts (although – similar to recall – state and physical context shifts may well affect the 'explicit recollection' component of recognition memory that we considered previously).

Unconscious influences on memory

Even in the absence of recall, recognition or feelings of familiarity, memory may still be observable. As we noted in Chapter 2, if information has been previously encountered, subsequent encounters with the same information may be different due to the previous encounter – even in the absence of any overt signs of memory. But unconscious effects of memory may be problematic. For example, formal studies have examined whether people are likely to believe assertions such as 'The tallest statue in the world is in Tibet', even when these assertions are untrue. It was found that people were more likely to believe these assertions if they had been encountered in a previous memory experiment – even if people could not remember these assertions in any other way. These unconscious effects of memory may be responsible for the effectiveness in a social context of some behavioural methods, such as propaganda.

As we saw in Chapter 2, *priming* describes the (often unconscious) behavioural influence on us of a past event. It can be measured by comparing behaviour following some event with the behaviour that arises if that event did not occur. In the above example, belief in specific assertions (for example, about the location of the world's largest statue) may be primed by having previously encountered these assertions. If two groups of people are compared – comprising some people who encountered an assertion, and some people who did not – the difference in beliefs is likely to represent a measure of the degree of priming from the earlier encounter. Here is another example of priming. Consider the word fragment '_i_c_o_e'. A researcher might measure how long it takes people to solve or complete the fragment to make a real English word (i.e. to say 'disclose'), and then compare the time taken by a) people who have recently encountered the word or idea with the time required by b) people who have not. Even when people have recently encountered the word 'disclose' but do not remember the experience of doing so, they can generally solve the word fragment more quickly than people who have not had this prior experience. (And, as we saw in Chapter 2, people with amnesia can perform this type of task well.) The difference in the time needed to respond to the cue is an example of priming – one type of evidence for memory (i.e. an enduring effect) of the previous experience.

Categories versus continuum?

We might consider the behaviours from which memory is inferred as existing along a continuum: free recall ... cued recall ... recognition ... feeling of familiarity ... unconscious behavioural influence. This view suggests that differences among these various manifestations of memory are due to the memories having different strengths or different availability. It would follow from this position that where memory is strong and available, free recall is possible – along with all of the other demonstrations of memory. But as memory weakens, or is otherwise less available, free recall would not occur – but memory might still be observable at 'lower' strengths or levels of availability (i.e. recognition, familiarity, unconscious influence).

This approach is appealing in its simplicity, but there are potential difficulties with a simple continuum approach. For example, the ability to recall information does not always mean that the information will be correctly recognized. Furthermore, some variables have the opposite effect on recognition and recall performance, such as word frequency. Frequently used words, such as 'table', are better recalled than lower frequency words like 'anchor'. However, the lower frequency words are better recognized. In addition, information that has been intentionally learned is generally better recalled than information that was acquired incidentally, but information that is learned unintentionally is sometimes better recognized. The key point here is that different (and, perhaps, unexpected) outcomes may be obtained on specific memory parameters when memory encoding is directly manipulated, indicating that memory effects are not mediated by a single straightforward system or process operating along a single continuum.

Relating study and test

As we have seen in this chapter, what we are able to retrieve depends largely on the context in which the information was encoded or classified in the first place, and to what extent this matches the retrieval context. We noted that Tulving developed the *encoding specificity principle*, emphasizing the relationship between what occurs at study time (encoding) and what occurs at test time (retrieval). What is encoded in any particular encoding situation is selective, i.e. it is determined by the demands on the individual at study time. According to Tulving, what will be remembered later depends on the similarity between the memory test conditions and the original study conditions. We saw an example of this when considering the experiments of Godden and Baddeley with divers tested on shore or underwater.

A further experiment conducted by Barclay and colleagues illustrates encoding specificity in more detail. These researchers required participants to study a series of sentences with key words embedded in the sentences. So, for example, the word 'PIANO' was presented in one of two sentences: 'The man tuned the PIANO' or 'The man lifted the PIANO'. At recall, the sentences were cued by phrases that were either a) appropriate or b) inappropriate to the particular attributes of the named object (the piano). When tested, participants who had received the sentence about tuning the piano being remembered 'PIANO' when they were cued with the phrase 'something melodious'. (According to the encoding specificity principle, this is because – for this group – the melodious aspect of the piano had not been emphasized in the sentence at the time of study.) Conversely, participants who had studied the sentence about lifting the piano at the time of encoding were more effectively cued at test by the phrase 'something heavy' rather than by the cue 'something melodious'. (By the encoding specificity principle, this is because – for this group – the weight aspect of the piano had been emphasized in the sentence at the time of study).

This experiment demonstrates two important aspects of encoding specificity:

1. Only those elements of the original event that are specifically activated by the study situation are certain to be encoded.
2. For information to be optimally recalled, test cues need to target the particular aspects of the information that were originally encoded. In other words, remembering depends on the match between what is encoded and what is cued.

So, to achieve the best recall, the type of processing involved when studying needs to be appropriately matched to the type of processing that will required at test. Morris and colleagues demonstrated the effect of *transfer appropriate processing* in an extension of the Craik and Tulving 'levels of processing' experiments that were referred to in Chapter 2. In the original Craik and Tulving studies, participants were encouraged during encoding to focus on the i) physical, ii) phonological (e.g. rhyming), or iii) semantic aspects of the to-be-remembered word. As we saw in Chapter 2, under typical testing conditions semantic processing during encoding led to the best level of recall during testing. But in a study conducted by Morris and colleagues, another condition was added in the test phase, whereby participants had to identify words that rhymed with the words presented earlier during encoding. For this new 'rhyming' retrieval condition, there was a closer match between i) the rhyming task during learning condition and ii) the rhyming match required at the time of the response. At test, the best recall of rhyming words was observed in participants where rhyming (i.e. phonological processing) had been the focus of the learning task. This finding again demonstrates the importance of the relationship between what is encoded and what is cued – one of the fundamental tenet of encoding specificity.

Chapter 4
Inaccuracies in memory

In this chapter, the question will be addressed of what underlies forgetting. The debate over whether we ever truly forget anything – or instead encounter difficulties retrieving stored information – will be considered. Other kinds of memory difficulty will also be discussed; for example, distortions and biases in memory induced by suggestion – the focus of a considerable body of work conducted over the past several decades (especially with respect to research on eyewitness testimony). We will also consider situations in which memory may work in a qualitatively more efficient manner, i.e. in so-called 'flashbulb memory' situations where it has been argued that memories may be especially vivid (remembering the assassination of John F. Kennedy or the death of Diana, Princess of Wales, for example). Related to this issue, we will consider emotional events impacting upon memory functioning, for example in situations of perceived threat or reward where we tend to retain information more efficiently.

Forgetting

> Please to remember the Fifth of November, Gunpowder Treason
> and Plot. We know no reason why gunpowder treason should ever
> be forgot.
>
> Anonymous

> The existence of forgetting has never been proved: we only know
> that some things don't come to mind when we want them to.

Friedrich Nietzsche

Recall the tripartite, logically necessary distinction between encoding, storage, and retrieval introduced in Chapter 1. *Forgetting* can be defined as the loss of information that has been put into storage. Forgetting may occur not because of problems in retaining information in storage, *per se*, but because similar memories become confused and interfere with each other when we try to retrieve them. If we wish to understand how memory works fully, then we need to try to understand some of the factors that can influence the forgetting of information.

There are two traditional views of forgetting. One view argues that memory simply fades or decays away, just as objects in the physical environment might fade or erode or tarnish over time. This view represents a more *passive* conceptualization of forgetting and memory. The second view regards forgetting as a more *active* process. According to this perspective, there is no strong evidence for the passive fading of information in memory, but forgetting occurs because memory traces are disrupted, obscured or overlaid by other memories. In other words, forgetting occurs as a consequence of interference.

The consensus in the current literature is that both of these processes occur, but it is often quite difficult to separate the importance of time – i.e. the fading away or decay of memories – from interference through other events, because often these two things occur together. For example, if you try to remember what happened in the Wimbledon Men's Tennis Final in 1995, your memory may be imperfect (a) because of forgetting due to the passage of time, (b) because of forgetting due to your memories of other intervening Wimbledon Men's Tennis Finals interfering with your memory of the 1995 final, or (c) because *both processes are operating together*. However, there is some evidence that interference may be the more important mechanism underlying forgetting (in other words, if you had not seen another tennis match since the Wimbledon Men's Tennis Final in 1995, then you might remember this event better than someone who had seen other tennis matches over the same period of time, because your memory for the 1995 Final is somehow more 'distinctive').

More generally, our experiences do tend to interact in our memories and to run into one another, with the result that our memory for one experience is often interrelated to our memory of another. The more similar two experiences are, the greater the likelihood that they will interact in our memory. In some cases, this interaction can be helpful in that new semantic learning can build on old learning (for example, there is evidence that chess experts can remember chess positions better than novices – as considered later in this chapter). But when it is important to separate two episodes and render them quite distinct, interference can mean that we remember less accurately than we would otherwise have done. For example, memories from two different Wimbledon tennis finals might become confused with one another.

Flashbulb memories and the reminiscence bump

One interesting feature of memory is that people seem to be able to remember certain events very vividly for a long time, especially if they are particularly unusual and arousing. Two different aspects of this phenomenon are i) *flashbulb memories* and ii) the *reminiscence bump*.

The assassination of John F. Kennedy in 1963, the death of Princess Diana in 1997, and the destruction of the Word Trade Centre in New York in 2001 are very memorable events for people who were alive when these events occurred. Memory for such events appears to be very resistant to forgetting over time. Many people are able to remember where they were and who they were with when they heard the news of one or all of these events. This is an example of what has been termed *flashbulb memory*. In highly arousing situations such as these, people often seem to remember well. This phenomenon may well be related to pressures operating during our evolutionary past. As stated by Shakespeare in *Henry V* when making reference to the Battle of Agincourt: 'Old men forget: yet all shall be forgot, But he'll remember with advantages what feats he did that day.'

By comparison, the *reminiscence bump* occurs when people are asked during later life to remember events from across their lifespan. In these situations, people tend to remember disproportionately more events from the period between their adolescence and early adulthood. This point was neatly encapsulated by the writer and lawyer John Mortimer when he stated that: 'The distant past, when I was acting my solo version of Hamlet before the blind eyes of my father, duelling with myself and drinking my own poisoned chalice ... seems as clear as yesterday. What are lost in the mists of vanishing memory are the events of ten years ago.' It has been suggested that this reminiscence bump is due to the particular significance of events that are occurring during the earlier portion of one's life. These are frequently events in which emotions are heavily involved (a consideration that may also be relevant for flashbulb memories). Such events include: meeting one's partner, getting married or becoming a parent – and events that are significant in other ways, such as starting work, graduating from university or backpacking around the world.

The areas of flashbulb memories and the reminiscence bump are both quite controversial; for example, with respect to flashbulb memories, it has been questioned to what extent semantic memory may intrude upon episodic memory for events such as the death of Princess Diana (such that we feel that we are remembering

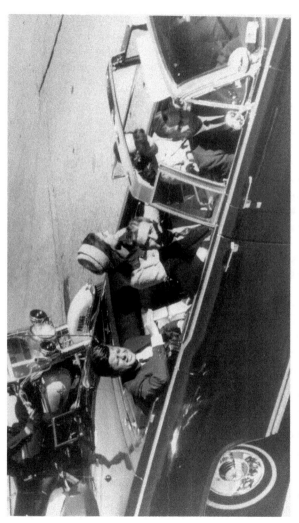

8. The assassination of John F. Kennedy in 1963, the death of Princess Diana in 1997, and the destruction of the Word Trade Centre in New York in 2001 are very memorable events for people who were alive when these events occurred

episodic detail richly, when in fact much of this detail may be inferred – refer to Chapter 2 for a brief consideration of the extent to which semantic and episodic memory may interact, and to Chapter 1 regarding the degree to which 'top down' influences may be relevant in memory). Nevertheless, both of these topics are the subjects of considerable interest in the memory literature.

Organization and errors in memory

The palest ink is better than the best memory.

Chinese proverb

In the 1960s and 1970s, some studies were carried out on chess players to find out how well they could remember the positions of chess pieces on a board. The studies showed that chess masters could remember 95% of the pieces on the chessboard after a single 5-second glance. But weaker chess players were able to position only 40% of the pieces correctly, and needed eight attempts to reach 95% correct performance. Examined in more detail, the findings suggested that the advantage enjoyed by the chess masters stemmed from their ability to perceive the chessboard as an organized whole, rather than as a collection of individual pieces. Similar effects have been shown with expert bridge players when they attempt to recall bridge hands, or where electronics experts are asked to remember electronic circuits. In each case, it appears that the experts organize the material into a coherent and meaningful pattern. Drawing on a rich background of prior experience, experts seem to be able to enhance their memory performance significantly above that of non-experts.

We have already seen in Chapter 3 that organizing information at the time of *retrieval* (in the form of cueing) can aid recall, but these studies of experts reveal the benefits of organization at the time of *learning* too. In the laboratory, researchers have compared memory for the learning of a) relatively unstructured material with the recall of b) material that had some structure imposed at

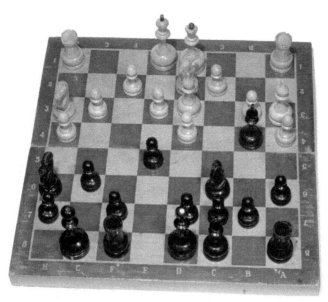

9. There is evidence that chess experts can remember chess positions better than novices. This is related to apparently the ability of experts to perceive the chessboard as an organized whole, rather than as a collection of individual pieces

the time of learning. For example, memory for a random list of words can be compared with memory for a list that has been segmented, for the purposes of presentation, into categories of, say, i) vegetables or ii) items of furniture at encoding. When people are asked to remember later the list that was organized during encoding, their performance is substantially better than when they heard the randomly organized list during the learning phase. Therefore, meaningful organization of information during learning can sometimes lead to enhanced memory performance at test. However, as we will see shortly, other types of organization during learning can result in distortions in memory when people are tested later.

The effects of previous knowledge

Schemas – what we already know

As we saw in Chapter 1, in the 1930s Bartlett asked English participants to read and then recall a Native American folk tale, *The War of the Ghosts*, which came from a culture that was very different from their own. When people attempted to recall this story, their reports were obviously based on the original tale, but they had inserted, deleted, and modified information to produce stories that seemed more sensible to them – what Bartlett termed an 'effort after meaning'.

Bartlett proposed that we possess *schemata* (or *schemas*), which he described as active organizations of past experiences. These schemas help us to make sense of familiar situations, guiding our expectations and providing a framework within which new information is processed. For example, we might possess a schema for a 'typical' day at work or at school, or for a 'typical' visit to a restaurant or to the cinema.

People seemingly have trouble understanding presented information if they cannot draw upon schemas for previously acquired knowledge. This point was nicely illustrated in a study conducted by Bransford and Johnson. These researchers gave participants a passage to remember, which began as follows:

> The procedure is actually quite simple. First you arrange items into different groups. Of course one pile may be sufficient depending on how much there is to do. If you have to go somewhere else due to lack of facilities that is the next step; otherwise you are pretty well set. It is important not to overdo things. That is, it is better to do too few things at once than too many.

Recalling this passage of text proved to be difficult for participants, even if the title of the piece was given after the passage had been read. Bransford and Johnson found that it was only when the title of the piece ('Washing Clothes') was given *in advance* of the text that subsequent recall was improved. With the title provided beforehand, the passage became more meaningful, and recall performance doubled. The explanation offered for these findings was as follows: providing the title in advance i) explained what the passage was about, ii) cued a familiar schema, and iii) helped people to make sense of the given statements. So it seems that providing a meaningful context improves memory.

It is possible to remember without understanding, though – especially with extra aids provided, such as having the information presented for verification using recognition testing (see Chapter 3). Alba and colleagues demonstrated that, although *recall* of the 'Washing Clothes' passage (referred to in the previous section) was much improved when the title was known in advance, *recognition* of sentences from the passage was equivalent, with or without the title. Alba and colleagues concluded that provision of the title allowed the participants to integrate the sentences into a more coherent unit, which benefited recall – but that this affected only the associations among the sentences, not the encoding of the sentences themselves (which is why recognition performance for the text material was apparently preserved, without provision of the title).

The research conducted with the 'washing clothes' passage illustrates how our previous knowledge helps us to remember information. Bower, Winzenz, and colleagues provided another demonstration. They asked participants to learn sets of words that were presented either a) randomly or b) in a well-organized hierarchy. These researchers found that presenting the words in meaningful hierarchies reduced the learning time to a quarter of that required for the same words when they were randomly positioned. The organization of the hierarchy apparently emphasized nuances of the words' meanings, which appeared not only to simplify the learning of the lists, but also to provide a framework within which the participants could structure their subsequent recall. So organization of memory material may work to enhance *both* i) learning and ii) recall for the same materials.

How does knowledge promote remembering?

As was indicated in Chapter 3, experts in any area find it easier and quicker to learn new information within their expertise than do novices. This finding indicates that what we learn appears to depend heavily on our existing knowledge. For example, Morris and colleagues showed that there was a very strong relationship between how much their participants knew about football and the number of new football scores they could remember after hearing them just once. Participants were read a new set of football scores as they were being broadcast at the weekend. One set of football scores were the real scores, while another set of scores was simulated by constructing plausible pairs of teams and assigning goals with the same frequency as had occurred in an earlier week. Participants in the study were told whether the scores they heard were real or simulated. Only the real scores seemed to activate the knowledge and interest of the football experts. For real scores, level of memory recall was clearly related to football expertise – so more knowledgeable fans recalled more of the scores. But for simulated scores (where the scores were highly plausible but not the genuine results), it was found that expertise had relatively little effect on subsequent recall performance. These findings illustrate the interaction of memory capacity with existing knowledge (and, presumably, interest and motivation, too) in determining what is effectively remembered.

How can knowledge lead to errors?

Our previous knowledge is a very valuable asset, but it can also lead to errors. In one relevant study, Owens and colleagues gave their participants a description of the activities performed by a particular character. For example, one of the sketches was about a student named Nancy. Here is the first part of that sketch:

Nancy went to the doctor. She arrived at the office and checked in with the receptionist. She went to see the nurse who went through the usual procedures. Then Nancy stepped on the scale and the nurse recorded her weight. The doctor entered the room and examined the results. He smiled at Nancy and said, 'Well, it seems my expectations have been confirmed.' When the examination was finished, Nancy left the office.

Half of the participants were told in advance that Nancy was worried that she was pregnant. These participants included between two and four times as many pieces of incorrect information when tested on their recall of the sketch. For example, some of them recalled the 'usual procedures' that were conducted as comprising 'pregnancy tests'. These types of errors were made in both recognition and recall tests. These findings reflect the fact that people have many expectations about how conventional activities (going to the doctor, a lecture, a restaurant) will proceed – and these expectations provide schemas that can either facilitate or mislead with respect to our memory functioning. In another part of their 'washing clothes' study, Bower and colleagues studied the influence of such schemas on subsequent recall. They gave their participants stories based on normal expectations, but the stories included significant variations from the norm. So, for example, a story about eating in a restaurant might refer to paying the bill at the beginning of the meal. When recalling the stories, participants tended to reorder their recall back to the schematic (i.e. more typical) form of the story. Other common errors that people made involved including actions that would normally be expected in that particular context, but which had not been mentioned in the original story – such as looking at the menu before selecting one's meal.

In general, the findings of these and similar studies indicate that people tend to remember what is consistent with their schemas, but filter out what is inconsistent.

Real versus imagined memories

As was mentioned in Chapter 1, even when we believe that we are literally 'playing back' some previous event or information in our mind, as if it were a videotape, we are actually constructing a memory from bits and pieces that we actually remember, along with our general (i.e. semantic) knowledge about how these bits should be assembled.

This strategy is usually very adaptive, minimizing our need to remember new things that are very similar to things we already know. But sometimes there can be a blurring between what actually happened and what has been imagined or suggested.

Reality monitoring

The issue of reality monitoring – i.e. identifying which memories are of real events, and which are of dreams or other imaginary sources – has been systematically addressed over a number of years by Marcia Johnson and her colleagues. Johnson has argued that qualitative differences between memories are important for distinguishing *external memories* from *internally generated* ones. She contends that external memories i) have stronger sensory attributes, ii) are more detailed and complex, and iii) are set in a coherent context of time and place. By contrast, Johnson argues that internally generated memories embody more traces of the reasoning and imagining processes that generated them.

Although Johnson found support for these differences, applying these proposed distinctions as defining criteria can nevertheless lead to our accepting some memories as real, even when they are not. For example, a study was conducted in the 1990s in which participants were required to recall details from a videotape, and to report both a) their confidence and b) the presence or absence of clear mental imagery and detail. Clear images and details were found to occur more often with correct reports of what had been presented on the videotape. However, the presence of accessible images led people to be overly confident, so that incorrect details accompanied by mental images were reported with greater confidence than correct details that lacked these associated images. These findings seem to indicate there is no completely reliable way of distinguishing between 'real' and 'imagined' memories.

Related to the concept of reality monitoring is *source monitoring* – i.e. being able to successfully attribute the origin of our memories (e.g. being able to state that we heard a particular piece of information a) from a friend rather than b) hearing it on the radio). As we shall see, errors in attributing memories can have important consequences – for example, during eyewitness testimony (Mitchell and Johnson, 2000).

Eyewitness testimony

Even aspects of our everyday environment can be very poorly remembered. For instance, in Chapter 1 we saw that it can be challenging to remember correctly something as straightforward as whether the head on a coin in one's pocket is pointing to the left or to the right. Generally speaking, people are very poor at answering this question, even when they use those particular coins almost every day. Some people might argue, though, that when we observe an *unusual* event (such as a crime), we are in a much better position to remember this effectively than when we are trying to remember the mundane features of a coin. After all, in our everyday lives we don't need to know which way the head points in order to be able to use coins effectively.

However, in a crime situation, we know that many factors work against an eyewitness, and can obscure or distort his or her memory:

- Although enhanced arousal can facilitate memory (as we have seen earlier), when a person is experiencing *extreme stress*, their attention can be narrowed (for example, towards a potentially dangerous weapon) and perception is often biased.

- Related to this last point, people tend to remember more poorly when they are in a *violent situation* – where self preservation is more the priority (for example, one may be allocating one's cognitive resources towards finding an exit route, or finding an item with which one could defend oneself – rather than towards processing the appearance and identity of the perpetrator).

- Associated with the above, a *weapon* located at the scene of a crime can distract a person's attention away from the perpetrator of the crime.

- Although we are much better at *recognizing* faces than *recalling* information, clothing is a particularly powerful source of bias in recognition – so an individual who happens to be wearing similar clothing to the culprit could be incorrectly 'identified'.

- People tend to be poorer at recognizing faces of individuals from *different racial and ethnic groups* to themselves – even when they have considerable experience of interacting with people from other races (furthermore, this phenomenon doesn't seem to be related to degree of racial prejudice).

Another powerful influence in the distortion of memory is the use of leading questions. 'Did you see *the man who raped* the woman?' is an example of a leading question. It can result in far more confirmations of an alleged crime than a question such as 'Did you see *a man rape* the woman?' So, suppose you witness an accident at a traffic junction, and you are later asked whether the car stopped before or after the tree. Asked such a question, you are subsequently likely to 'insert' a tree into my memory of the scene, even if there was no tree there in the first place. And once the tree has been inserted, it tends to operate as if it were part of the original memory, so that it is difficult to tell the difference between the real memory and what has been subsequently introduced.

One particularly salient example of memory bias was experienced by Donald Thompson, who (ironically, as we shall see) had been very active in arguing for the unreliability of eyewitness evidence.

On one occasion, Thompson took part in a television debate on the very topic of eye-witness testimony. Some time later, the police arrested him, but declined to explain why. It was only after a woman picked him out of a line-up at the police station that he discovered he was to be charged with rape. When he asked for further details, it became clear that the rape had been committed at the same time as he'd been taking part in the television discussion. So he had a very good alibi (of course) with a large number of witnesses, including a police officer taking part in the same discussion! It seemed that, coincidentally, the woman had been raped while this television program was being broadcast in the room in which her rape was committed. This represented a problem with source monitoring, also called 'source amnesia' (or what Dan Schacter, among his 'Seven Sins of Memory', has called *misattribution*; please see Further reading on page 139). So it appeared that the woman's memory of the rapist had been contaminated by the face (of Donald Thompson) that she saw on the television at the same time. (The topic of discussion in the TV programme may also have been highly relevant.) So the woman recognized Thompson's face, but the source of the recognition was misattributed.

On a related topic, other studies have reported situations in which people have been unable to recognize when two people have changed places. This is a phenomenon referred to as 'change blindness', where people are apparently quite poor at judging whether a change has taken place in their immediate environment. Taken together with problems that can arise with eyewitness testimony, change blindness indicates how vulnerable we can be with respect to the inaccurate processing of some information in our immediate environment.

The misinformation effect

The distortion of memory through the incorporation of new information has been an important research topic for researchers concerned both with the practical implications for eyewitness testimony, and with theoretical accounts of the nature of memory. Despite what we know about the fallibilities of memory, considerable weight is typically still placed on eyewitness testimony by the legal profession, the police and the press. But (as we have see in the previous section) eyewitnesses may be expected to produce 'information' that is quite unrealistic in the context of what we know – from carefully conducted scientific experiments – about the way our memories work. Eyewitnesses' reports of crimes may also depend on their emotional investment and their personal perspective; for example, whether they are more sympathetic towards the perpetrator of the crime or towards the victim.

Elizabeth Loftus and her colleagues have explored in depth the *misinformation effect*. Specifically, Loftus and colleagues have repeatedly demonstrated distortions of memory after intervening, misleading questioning or information. This issue arises when misleading information is introduced indirectly. For example, Loftus and colleagues showed participants a series of slides along with the story of a road traffic accident. Later, the participants were questioned about the event. One of the questions was slightly different for half of the participants, in that it referred to a 'Stop' sign instead of a 'Yield' ('Give Way') sign. Participants who were asked a question with misleading information included within it were more likely to affirm that false information in a later recognition memory test. These participants tended to choose the road sign that had been mentioned in the misleading question, rather than the one they had actually seen. The findings are robust and have important implications for the sort of questions that eyewitnesses of crimes and accidents should be asked if their recall is to be as accurate as possible. However, the basis of the misinformation effect continues to be disputed by some researchers. Those who challenge Loftus' interpretation of her findings argue it is indeed possible that the participants' original memories are permanently distorted by the questioning, but it is also possible that the questions merely supplement participants' memories by providing information that the participants would not otherwise be able to remember. This issue will be discussed further later in this chapter.

Overall, however, the central message from these studies is, once more, that memory should not be regarded as a passive process: as we saw in Chapter 1, it is a 'top-down' system influenced by our 'mental set' (our preconceptions, stereotypes, beliefs, attitudes, and thoughts) as well as a 'bottom-up' system influenced by sensory input. In other words, memory isn't solely driven by sensory information derived from our physical environment, with people passively receiving that information and putting it into their memory wholesale. Rather, influenced by our past knowledge and presuppositions, we impose meaning on perceived information, biasing our memories to be consistent with our general world view.

False memories

Related to the misinformation effect, but with more potentially serious consequences, are recovered and false memories. Under therapy, some adults have 'recovered' memories of alleged abuse in childhood that have led to criminal convictions. But in these situations are people truly 'recovering' memories of genuine events that occurred during their childhood, or are they being induced to remember things that didn't actually happen? Substantial research has shown that, under certain circumstances, false memories can be created. Sometimes these are benign – for example, Roediger, McDermott and colleagues have conducted an extensive body of research since the 1990s showing that people can be encouraged to 'remember' an item that is semantically linked to a series of previously presented items, but which itself was not presented (for example, people may come to

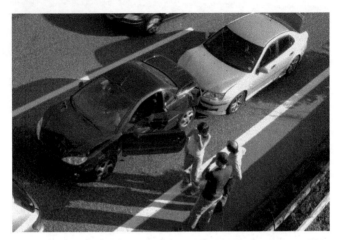

10. Our memory for events such as a car accident can be influenced by the kind of question we are asked, such that information can be 'inserted' into our memory. This phenomenon – known as the misinformation effect – has profound implications for eyewitness testimony

remember having been presented with the word 'night', when they were previously presented with a series of words that are semantically associated with 'night', such as 'dark', 'moon', 'black', 'still', 'day' ...).

Less benignly, it is also possible to create – using suggestions and misleading information – memories for 'events' that the individual believes very strongly happened in their past but which are, in fact, false. So it remains at least plausible that some abusive events that people 'remember' are in fact false memories.

In her laboratory experiments, Elizabeth Loftus found that people respond just as rapidly and confidently to misleading questions as they do to questions phrased without bias. In such situations, even if the participant notices that new information has been introduced, this can still become part of their 'memory' of the incident – so memory bias can be introduced retrospectively (even if it is consciously identified as such). In one experiment, Loftus and Palmer asked some students to watch a series of films, each showing a traffic accident. Afterwards they had to answer questions about the events. One of the questions was: 'How fast were the cars going when they ------- each other?' The gap was filled with a different word for each group of students, and could be any one of the following: 'smashed', 'collided', 'bumped', 'hit' or 'contacted'. What the researchers found was that the students' estimates of the speed of the cars was influenced by the choice of verb in that particular question. Loftus and Palmer concluded that the students' memory of the accident had been altered by the implied information provided in the question.

Loftus and Palmer went on to research this issue further by asking students to watch a film of a multiple-car accident. Again, the students were asked about the speed of the cars, with the word 'smashed' (implying greater collision speed) being used for one group of students and 'hit' for another. A third group of students weren't asked this particular question. A week later, the students were asked to answer more questions, one of which was 'Did you see any broken glass?' at the scene of the accident.

Loftus and Palmer found that not only did the verb used in the speed question influence the students' estimates of speed, but that this question subsequently influenced their answer to the broken glass question that was posed a week later. So, those students who had estimated a higher speed were more likely to remember seeing broken glass at the scene of the accident – although there hadn't, in fact, been any broken glass in the film. Those students who hadn't been asked the speed question previously were least likely to remember seeing broken glass, when asked about this a week later.

In another study, Loftus again showed participants a film of a traffic accident. This time she asked some of the participants:

'How fast was the white sports car going when it passed the barn while travelling along the country road?' In fact, there had been no barn in the film. A week later, those participants who had been asked this question were more likely to say they remembered seeing a barn in the film. Even if participants were asked simply 'Did you see a barn?' shortly after viewing the film, they were more likely – a week later – to 'remember' seeing it.

Loftus concluded from these results that the memory representation of an event can be changed by the subsequent introduction of misleading information. Some researchers have argued, however, that participants in these studies were simply conforming to what was expected of them – just as a child will give the answer they think is expected of them, rather than say that they 'don't know'. However, Loftus proceeded to find more convincing evidence to support her conclusion.

Memory

Loftus and colleagues again presented participants with a traffic accident, but this time it was on a series of slides. The accident showed a red Datsun turning at an intersection and hitting a pedestrian, but one group of participants i) saw the car stopping first at a 'Stop' sign, while another group ii) saw it stopping at a 'Yield' sign. The critical question this time was: 'Did another car pass the red Datsun while it was stopped at the Stop sign?' or 'Did another car pass the red Datsun while it was stopped at the Yield sign?'. For half the participants from each group, the word 'Stop' was used, and for the other half of the participants from each group, 'Yield' was used. Half of the participants in each group received information that was consistent with what they had seen in the accident, and the other half of each group received misleading information.

Twenty minutes later, all the participants were shown pairs of slides, where one of each pair of slides showed what they had actually seen and the other was slightly different. The participants had to choose the most accurate slide for each pair. One of the pairs showed the car halting at a 'Stop' sign, while the other slide showed it halting at a 'Yield' sign. The researchers found that those participants who had been asked the question earlier that had been consistent with what they had seen in the original slides were more likely to choose the correct slide when they were asked to choose the most accurate slide, twenty minutes later. By contrast, those participants who had been asked a misleading question earlier were more likely to choose the wrong slide when they were asked to choose the most accurate slide, twenty minutes later. Although somewhat complicated to evaluate, this finding suggests that some people were actually *remembering* according to the information that had been introduced concerning the 'Stop' or 'Yield' sign after the event, rather than simply conforming to what was expected of them – as some of Loftus' opponents had previously suggested (because each participant now had two, equally plausible responses to choose from at the time of test).

These findings have great significance for interviewing techniques undertaken by police officers, lawyers, judges and other workers in the judicial system. Conversely, some other findings suggest that, under certain conditions, memory can operate in such a way that subsequent relevant information is inappropriately *not* incorporated (as it should be). This complementary body of research indicates that, although people may remember corrections to earlier misinformation, they may nevertheless continue to rely on the discredited information (as observed in laboratory investigations conducted by Lewandowsky and colleagues). With respect to real world examples of this phenomenon, consider the following: approximately one year after the invasion of Iraq in 2003, 30% of respondents in a US survey still believed that weapons of mass destruction had been found in the country. And several months after President George Bush declared the war against Iraq to have ended (in May 2003), 20% of Americans believed that Iraq had used chemical or biological weapons on the battlefield during the conflict. Therefore, in

'The Seven Sins of Memory', proposed by Dan Schacter

Dan Schacter has proposed that memory's malfunctions can be divided into seven fundamental transgressions or 'sins':

absent-mindedness: a breakdown at the interface between attention and memory – rather than losing information over time, we either did not register the information in the first place, or we don't look for it when it is needed, because our attention is focused elsewhere;

transience: a weakening or loss of memory over time – so we can remember what we did today, but in a few months' time we will most likely have forgotten it due to decay;

blocking: a thwarted search for information that we may be desperately trying to retrieve – the 'tip of the tongue phenomenon' is an example of this malfunction;

misattribution: assigning memory to the wrong source – so you might hear about something on the TV, but later wrongly remember the information as having been passed on by a colleague at work;

suggestibility: memories that are implanted as a result of leading questions, comments or suggestions – together with misattribution, this can cause serious problems in a forensic context;

bias: the powerful influence of our current knowledge and beliefs on how we remember our pasts – so we unconsciously distort past events or learned material in the light of our current perspective, and in our attempts to present ourselves in a positive light to others;

persistence: repeated recall of disturbing information or events that we would prefer to banish from our minds – this could range from an embarrassing blunder at work to a seriously traumatic experience (as in post-traumatic stress disorder).

some situations, there appears to be a retention of incorrect information in memory – a phenomenon which can also have profound social consequences. Characterizing further the environmental conditions which predispose towards either i) erroneous retrospective bias of memory (identified by Loftus and colleagues) or ii) inappropriate failure to incorporate relevant information presented after the original event (identified by Lewandowsky and colleagues) represents an important challenge for future research.

Chapter 5
Memory impairment

This chapter will consider the condition of memory loss, or 'amnesia' – when memory does not work effectively due to brain injury. With reference to the different subcomponents of memory that were discussed in previous chapters, the focus here will be on the loss of memory in the so-called classical amnesic syndrome. Relevant metaphors will be considered with respect to long-term memory functioning, incorporating the broad working distinction between the 'printing press' (which creates new long-term memories) and the 'library' (which stores older, 'consolidated' long-term memories). Much has been learned about the normal workings of memory through the study of individuals with damaged memory due to brain injury, and this chapter will provide an overview of these important findings. This chapter will also consider how other clinical conditions and mental states can influence memory.

Memory and the brain

So far in this book, we have been primarily considering memory in terms of its functional components and processes – the 'software' of memory, so to speak. But we can also think about memory at another level – in terms of the 'hardware' of the central nervous system that mediates memory. Deep within our brains, memories are sorted (or consolidated) in a part of the brain called the *hippocampus,* which acts as the 'printing press' for new memories. Important memories are 'printed' by the hippocampus, and then filed away (as 'books') indefinitely in the *cerebral cortex.* The cortex is the outer layer of the brain, where a vine-like thicket of billions of nerve cells reverberates via electrical and chemical impulses to retain information. The cerebral cortex may be regarded as the 'library', in which those important long-term memories ('books') that have been 'printed' by the hippocampus are stored indefinitely. (The degree to which the hippocampus

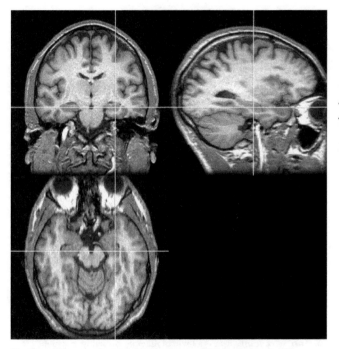

11. One of the most important structures of the brain involved in memory is the hippocampus, indicated by the cross hairs in the brain images, above

remains involved in retrieving these memories over longer time intervals remains – at the time of writing – contentious.)

Much research into memory has focused on what people do, say, feel, and imagine as a result of their previous experiences. But it is also important to consider how past events are reflected in our brain activity – especially in the context of clinical conditions that can impact adversely on memory. We now turn to a consideration of what can happen when the 'hardware' in the brain underlying memory becomes damaged.

Loss of memory after brain injury – the 'amnesic syndrome'

The amnesic syndrome is the purest example of memory impairment, involving some form of specific brain injury (typically involving those parts of the brain known as the *hippocampus* or the *diencephalon*). In the amnesic syndrome, patients exhibit a

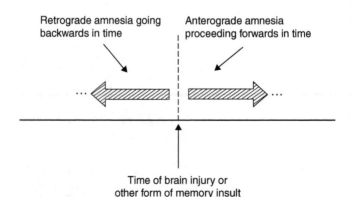

Retrograde amnesia going backwards in time

Anterograde amnesia proceeding forwards in time

Time of brain injury or other form of memory insult

12. *Anterograde amnesia* is a form of memory difficulty in which events or information presented after the time of injury cannot be remembered. By contrast, *retrograde amnesia* is a form of memory impairment in which someone is unable to remember information or events that were presented before the time of injury

severe *anterograde* amnesia and a degree of *retrograde* amnesia: anterograde amnesia refers to a loss of memory for information that occurred after the time of the brain injury that caused the memory loss, whereas retrograde amnesia refers to the loss of information occurring before the injury (see Figure 12).

Here is an account from a famous amnesic patient, NA, who was rendered amnesic after sustaining a very specific and quite unusual brain injury:

> I was working at my desk ... My room mate had come in [and] he had taken one of my small fencing foils off the wall and I guess he was making like Cyrano de Bergerac behind me ... I just felt a tap on the back ... I swung around ... at the same time he was making the lunge. I took it right in the left nostril, went up and punctured the cribriform area of my brain.

What follows is an excerpt from the interesting and revealing conversation that patient NA held with a psychologist, Wayne Wickelgren, who was introduced to NA in a room at the Massachusetts Institute of Technology (MIT) in the USA. NA heard Wickelgren's name and he said:

> 'Wickelgren, that's a German name isn't it?'
> Wickelgren said, 'No.'
> 'Irish?'
> 'No.'
> 'Scandinavian?'
> 'Yes, it's Scandinavian.'

There followed five minutes of further conversation between NA and Wickelgren, then Wickelgren left the room. Five minutes later, Wickelgren returned. NA apparently looked at Wickelgren as if he had never seen him before, and the two people were therefore reintroduced. The following conversation then ensued:

'Wickelgren, that's a German name isn't it?'

Wickelgren said, 'No.'

'Irish?'

'No.'

'Scandinavian?'

'Yes, it's Scandinavian.'

Note that – from the above account – not all types of memory are abolished in NA, as NA retains his knowledge of language; for example, he understood what was said to him, and he produced sensible verbal utterances. Related to this point, his semantic memory is at least partially preserved (see Chapter 2). In addition, NA's working memory abilities are sufficiently preserved for him to keep track of what is being said in the conversation. What NA seems to lack is *the specific ability to retain new information over any significant period of time.* In other words, he lacks the ability to put new information into long-term memory. This is one of the central characteristics of the amnesic syndrome.

More generally, in people with the amnesic syndrome, intelligence, language, and immediate memory span are maintained. But long-term memory is severely impaired. The nature of this impairment is a matter of considerable debate, with some theorists having argued that there is a selective loss of *episodic* memory in the amnesic syndrome (where episodic memory is defined as memory for the events of your life that you have experienced; see Chapter 2). By contrast, other researchers having argued for a wider ranging deficit in classical amnesia encompassing *declarative* memory (which refers to memory for facts, events or propositions that can be brought to mind and consciously expressed; it overlaps significantly with the concept of explicit memory, discussed in Chapter 2). By contrast, the amnesic syndrome appears to have little effect on procedural or implicit memory (such as remembering how to drive), and even

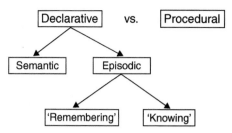

13. Squire proposed a model that differentiates within long-term memory between declarative (or explicit) memory versus procedural (or implicit) memory, with only declarative memory being compromised in the amnesic syndrome

new procedural memories can be formed effectively (that is, new skills or habits can be acquired effectively, such as – say – juggling or riding a monocycle).

The classical amnesic syndrome typically involves damage to the hippocampus and to closely connected brain regions such as the thalamus in the diencephalon. It therefore appears that damage to the hippocampus and the thalamus can prevent new conscious memories from being formed. Moreover, when individuals with amnesia learn new skills, they appear to achieve this without awareness. HM, who had had his hippocampus surgically removed, was eventually able to solve a complicated puzzle, called mirror drawing, that he attempted over many days (see figure 14). Yet, each time he was given the task to complete, he denied having ever seen this puzzle before!

This is a very important point when considering the way in which different aspects of memory *fractionate* or *dissociate* after brain injury, and may be useful when considering possible methods of rehabilitation for people with memory disorders. It can also tell us some important information about the way in which memory is organized in the healthy or non-damaged brain. Specifically, it has

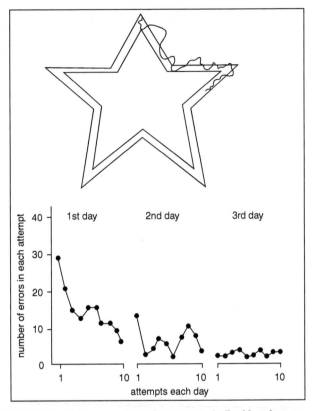

14. Patients with the amnesic syndrome are typically able to learn to perform a complicated task, called mirror drawing, attempted over several days – yet each time they are given the task to complete, they may well deny having ever undertaken the task before! (Individuals with amnesia typically perform normally, or very close to normally, on a wide range of implicit or procedural memory tasks)

been famously suggested (by Kenneth Craik) that, for complex systems such as the brain, we may learn more about the functional relationships in these systems i) when they cease to function properly rather than ii) when everything is working smoothly. Furthermore, as we saw in Chapter 2 several proposed functional distinctions in memory have been proposed in an attempt to understand findings that have been obtained in evaluating both a) healthy individuals and b) people with different forms of brain injury. Both of these sources of information have provided insightful findings pertaining to the organization of human memory.

On a related theme, there was a tendency in the past to categorize together all the different subtypes of amnesia according to whether an individual had an identifiable functional memory problem. But it is now apparent that different subtypes of amnesia have different characteristics, depending on the precise location of the brain damage. In future, we need to develop a more informed taxonomy of different memory-related brain disorders.

Making inferences about memory and the brain

The study of amnesia has been important in recent years as a) a way of discriminating between certain types of memory processes, and b) in linking deficits in remembering with specific neurological structures that are often damaged in patients with memory problems. In addition, the development of brain imaging techniques such as functional magnetic resonance imaging (fMRI) and positron emission tomography (PET) has added significant new *convergent* information by allowing us to study the parts of the brain that are active when non brain-damaged people remember. Brain imaging has also proven very useful for investigating a range of other clinical conditions and states in which different types of memory loss can be implicated, including (but not limited to) conditions as wide ranging as depression, stroke, post traumatic stress disorder, fatigue, schizophrenia, and déjà vu (see Chapter 3). There have even been some recent controversial suggestions that functional imaging can be used to evaluate the guilt or innocence of a potential criminal, by determining whether someone has a 'memory' for events and/or locations specifically associated with the crime.

But inferring generalizations about memory and the brain is difficult, because remembering is a complex process – involving many cognitive subcomponent processes (see previous chapters of this book) subserved by a constellation of brain mechanisms. That is, many parts of the brain are active when someone is remembering. This has been vividly illustrated by brain imaging studies conducted over the past several decades, implicating a host of brain regions that previously were not strongly associated with memory (such as the prefrontal cortex, located just above and behind the eyes, in encoding and retrieval). It is therefore challenging to seek to isolate neural activity that might be unique to remembering. This valid point notwithstanding, certain parts of the brain do seem to be important to memory, in particular.

Testing amnesia

Temporal lobe amnesic patients (such as HM in Boston or SJ, whom we have studied in Perth, Australia) have taught us a lot about the neurological basis of memory. In particular, it seems that important elements of long-term memory are served by the hippocampus, deep within the temporal lobe of the brain. Patient HM received surgery for the treatment of intractable epilepsy in 1953. The surgeon removed the inner face of the temporal lobe in each hemisphere, including parts of the hippocampus, the amygdala, and the rhinal cortex. Since this time, HM has remembered almost nothing new, though he still seems to remember some events in his life from before the surgical procedure. His other cognitive skills (e.g. intelligence, language, immediate memory span) seem to be unaffected. Furthermore, as we saw previously, people with the amnesic syndrome are capable of learning new motor skills, like mirror drawing (Figure 14), and perceptual skills like completing pictures – although he does not remember doing so.

Here is an example of a typical memory testing interview conducted with patients like HM. Before testing begins, HM introduces himself and talks with the neuropsychologist for a few minutes, having not met him before. The neuropsychologist asks HM what he had for breakfast that day: he does not remember. Systematic testing of memory then begins. The neuropsychologist removes a collection of photographs of faces from his briefcase. He shows some to HM, who studies them carefully. But a few minutes later, HM cannot identify which faces he has just seen and which ones he did not. His performance on this task is considerably lower than that of a comparison, control participant – who is of a similar age, gender, and background to HM, but who has not sustained brain damage. The same findings are obtained with a list of words that are read out aloud to HM, and which he is later asked to remember. The neuropsychologist then shows HM an elementary line drawing and asks him if he can identify it. HM correctly identifies this line drawing as a chair. He is also able to repeat a string of six numbers immediately after hearing them. The neuropsychologist leaves the room, and HM waits in the room, reading a magazine. Twenty minutes later, the neuropsychologist returns. HM clearly does not recognize the neuropsychologist: HM stands up, and politely introduces himself again. (We have obtained a similar pattern of findings in Western Australia with patient SJ.)

HM and SJ are both particularly 'pure' amnesic patients, i.e. they have a highly selective memory loss. SJ's brain damage is more confined to the hippocampus than HM's, but they appear to manifest similar clinical and test profiles. HM's and SJ's short-term memory is intact, but their memory for everyday events is disastrously impaired. It was initially suggested that HM's brain damage left him specifically unable to consolidate (i.e. store) new memories. However, since this time, it has been recognized that HM and other temporal lobe amnesic patients such as SJ can learn new skills and perform implicit memory tasks, as we have previously noted. It therefore seems unlikely that a straightforward consolidation failure can account for all of the symptoms in such individuals.

However, there is current controversy regarding the extent to which 'old' memories from before the time of the brain injury can be accessed by patients such as HM and SJ. So, more than fifty years after his surgery, neuroscientists still do not agree on exactly why HM shows his characteristic profound memory loss. Nonetheless, HM's case – and that of other similar patients with the amnesic syndrome – has focused considerable attention on the hippocampus as a core memory structure. This has proved to be a crucial step in increasing our knowledge concerning the 'hardware' of the brain underpinning memory, and in developing neuroscientific theories of information storage.

Amnesia has profound philosophical implications, given the degree to which our ongoing sense of personhood, self, and identity is intimately entwined with our memory. And at a practical level, memory loss is extremely debilitating given the range of everyday activities in which memory is important, and it can place great strain on carers. For example, it can be extremely frustrating for a carer to be asked the same question or to do the same thing over and over and over again, because someone can't remember having been asked the question or the task being done before. Some memory strategies have been found to be reliably effective for people with memory loss after brain injury, such as errorless learning techniques (see Chapter 7). External aids, such as personal organizers – which prompt people at certain times to do specific things – can help in cases of memory loss. But memory is not like a muscle that can be improved by repetitive exercise. So by remembering reams and reams of Shakespeare, you won't improve your general memory ability, unless in practising Shakespeare you devise more general memory strategies or techniques that can then be applied in other domains (such as using visual imagery; see Chapter 7).

Assessment of memory disorders

It is important in both clinical practice and research to carry out a range of systematic assessments of patients with memory disorders. Memory impairments sometimes occur in isolation, as in the case of HM, SJ or NA. But this is a very rare occurrence. For example, one of the more common forms of memory impairment is found in 'Korsakoff's syndrome', which usually affects other psychological capacities in addition to memory. Therefore, it is advisable to assess other mental abilities such as perception, attention, and intelligence – as well as language and executive functions – in someone who presents with memory loss.

For amnesic patients, psychologists often begin an assessment with the Wechsler Memory Scale (WMS, now in its third edition, the WMS-III). But other tests are also useful; for example, the Wechsler Adult Intelligence Scale (WAIS, also now in its third edition, the WAIS-III) might also be used, so that performance on the WAIS-III can be compared to that on the WMS-III. If there is a substantial difference between the WMS and WAIS scores, this indicates that the amnesic person has a particular impairment in memory – but not in 'intelligence' *per se*.

Intelligence should be assessed both currently using the WAIS (or a similar instrument) and premorbidly (using an indicator of IQ from before the illness), to determine if there has been any significant decline in intelligence over time, as a consequence of the clinical disorder.

Both the WAIS and WMS scales are periodically updated, and are standardized with respect to the healthy population. This is typical of most commercially available psychometric tests. So the WMS-III or the WAIS-III can be administered, and the results compared against the general population. The Wechsler test scales have been devised such that the mean of the general population is 100, with a standard deviation of 15. So anyone scoring 85 on the WAIS-III is scoring one standard deviation below the mean of the general population.

However, the assessment of memory provided by the WMS-III is not comprehensive, and other tests of memory and (if possible) other cognitive capacities should also be given when evaluating amnesia. These include assessment of remote and autobiographical memory. Clinical questionnaires about memory can also yield valuable information that psychometric measures do not necessarily provide – in particular, an important insight into the patient's everyday difficulties may be provided by the caregiver or by the patient themselves. Furthermore, although a memory impaired person may not be totally accurate in completing such questionnaires, one may be able to gain some insight into the patient's own perception of his or her memory functioning through the administration of such instruments.

As an overview of amnesia, note:

- new learning of information over a substantial time span may be impossible, even though people with amnesia can typically recite back normally information within their working memory span
- individuals with amnesia may well retain childhood memories, but typically find it almost impossible to acquire new memories – such as the names of people they just met
- amnesic people may well remember how to tell the time, but not remember what month, date or day it is currently, or be able to learn the layout of a new house
- people with amnesia may be able to learn new skills like typing; despite behavioural evidence of this new learning, they may deny having ever used a keyboard the next time they sit down to type!

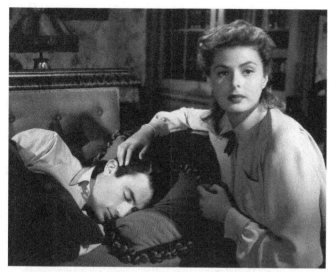

15. In the fugue state, someone apparently loses track of their personal identity and the memories that went with it. This condition may be caused by a traumatic event such as an accident or crime. Such a scenario is depicted in the film *Suspicion*, directed by Alfred Hitchcock

Psychogenic amnesia

Not all memory disorders result from organic illness or injury. In 'psychogenic amnesia', there is usually a functional impairment of memory, but no tangible evidence of neurological brain injury.

For example, there are instances of individuals entering a *dissociative state* when they seem to become partly or wholly separated from their memories. This is often caused by an event of a violent nature, such as physical or sexual abuse, or having committed or witnessed a murder. An example of a dissociative state is the fugue state, when someone loses track of their personal identity and the memories that went with it. Individuals experiencing a fugue state are usually unaware that anything is wrong, and will often adopt a new identity. The fugue only becomes apparent when the patient 'comes to', days, months, or even years after the precipitating event – often finding themselves some distance from where they were originally living (the term 'fugue' is, in fact, derived from the Latin for 'flight').

Another form of dissociative state is 'multiple personality disorder', in which a number of personalities apparently emerge to manage different aspects of an individual's past life. For example, in the case of the notorious Los Angeles Hillside Strangler in the late 1970s, Kenneth Bianchi was charged with the rape and murder of several women, but despite strong evidence against him, he persistently denied his guilt and claimed that he knew nothing about the crimes. Under hypnosis, however, another personality called 'Steve' emerged. 'Steve' was very different from 'Ken', and claimed responsibility for the murders. When removed from the hypnotic trance, Kenneth Bianchi could apparently remember nothing of the conversation between Steve and the hypnotist. If two or more personalities can exist within the same individual, this obviously creates significant legal problems in terms of which person should be charged with the crime! However, the ruling went against Bianchi in this case – because the court refused to accept that he genuinely possessed two different personalities.

In his trial, a number of psychologists pointed out that Bianchi's other personality emerged in hypnotic sessions – in which the examiner had actually suggested to Bianchi that he would reveal another part of himself. Hypnosis is itself a controversial technique, in terms of whether it can truly induce a qualitatively different state of consciousness. Furthermore, a specific issue here is whether the hypnotic effects were simply due to compliance with instructions given by the examiner – an issue analogous to one of the main issues under consideration with respect to many of Elizabeth Loftus' findings and their implications regarding the plausibility of eyewitness testimony (see Chapter 4). In the context of Bianchi, hypnosis may have allowed the suggestion that another personality could exist – and Bianchi may have seized the

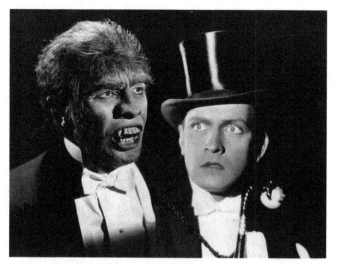

16. 'Multiple personality disorder' is a controversial dissociative state in which a number of personalities apparently emerge to deal with different aspects of an individual's life; a rather exaggerated version of this syndrome was depicted in the book *Dr Jekyll and Mr Hyde*

opportunity to confess via this conduit. Furthermore, Bianchi's general knowledge about psychiatric illness – together with his knowledge concerning previously reported cases of multiple personality – may have provided him with a basis for responding more veridically under hypnosis (i.e. at the time when the examiner had suggested to Bianchi that he would reveal another aspect of himself).

Because of its dramatic nature, so-called multiple personality disorder has been the subject of intense media interest, and a number of popular books describing individual cases have appeared. *The Three Faces of Eve* and (more recently) *Primal Fear* are two examples of successful films based on this rare disorder. In the more recent *Primal Fear*, the film portrays a man accused of murder successfully 'faking' multiple personality disorder, and being acquitted of the crime for which he was indeed responsible.

In everyday life, it seems that memory loss is indeed sometimes malingered or 'faked', and detection of malingering remains a challenge in a medicolegal context. By malingering or 'faking bad', we are here referring to an individual consciously performing at a lower level than that at which the same individual could perform if they were trying to the best of their ability. Less controversially, in recent times this phenomenon has been referred to as manifesting lowered (or reduced) effort – a more objective and less emotive term than malingering. The manifestation of reduced effort may be mediated consciously (e.g. for financial reward, or to generate increased attention from caregivers), or the motivation might be at a deeper unconscious level. Whatever the source of the motivation to 'fake bad', reliable techniques are fortunately now available to relevant professionals, enabling them to distinguish between those individuals with and without an objective memory impairment, and those that are exaggerating.

Chapter 6
The seven ages of man

Memory development

Referring back to the tripartite distinction between encoding, retention, and retrieval cited in Chapter 1, memory development can be regarded as the gradual emergence of more complex strategies for encoding and retrieving memories (with storage processes being relatively constant through development). This is especially the case as semantic knowledge increases and language becomes available. For example, there is evidence that increasing semantic knowledge enhances the way in which information in permanent memory can be accessed, and that the acquisition of language allows children to be able to encode materials more richly in terms of verbal labels – and use those labels as cues at retrieval. There is also evidence that the development of other cognitive skills can impact positively upon memory capacity; for example, the development of problem solving and hypothesis-testing skills may be relevant when trying to retrieve memories and when seeking to determine whether retrieved information is veridical.

With respect to explicit memory capacity, there is evidence of a graded emergence of full capacity – such that even young infants seem capable of recognition memory (for example, for the face of a caregiver), while rudimentary recall ability seems to be present by around five months of age. There is now an impressive body of evidence indicating that even pre-linguistic infants can manifest memory which is enduring and specific. These findings have been amassed using techniques which do not involve language, such as comparison, habituation, conditioning, and imitation – together with some techniques adapted from the non-human literature (such as delayed response and delayed non-matching to sample). Researchers such as Rovee-Collier have argued that the mechanisms underlying memory processes are fundamentally the same in infants and adults: information is forgotten gradually, recovered by reminders, and modified by new information that overlaps with previously information. However, as children mature memories are retrieved faster after longer delays, and via a range of different retrieval cues.

Studies of implicit memory (or memory without awareness; see Chapter 2) indicate that this may be intact in children as young as three years of age (for example, perceptual learning, verbal priming). Of note, this aspect of memory does not appear to show such a striking developmental improvement, perhaps related to this form of memory being mediated by evolutionarily longer established brain regions. In fact, there has been some suggestion that implicit memory doesn't improve much beyond childhood. By contrast, there seems to be a progressive development of meta-memory skills (i.e. knowledge about and regulation of memory processes), such that children develop a better awareness of how good or poor their memory is in particular situations, and how likely they are to be able to remember certain pieces of information. There is evidence of slightly later maturation of these capacities though (compared with what might be considered the 'core' memory of capacities of encoding, retention and retrieval). This is perhaps related to the relatively slow neural maturation of the frontal lobes of the brain through adolescence. As the name suggests, this is the part of the brain which occupies the front portion of the skull. (This brain region appears to have developed disproportionately in humans relative to other mammalian species.) We will discuss this brain region further, later in this chapter, in the context of ageing.

The question of what underlies memory development is yet to be fully answered. Children's state of knowledge and other abilities that may impact upon memory (such as their linguistic and visuo-spatial abilities) are undoubtedly important. But the neural maturation of the brain and other biological factors are likely to be critical too. One interesting aspect of children's memory, which remains rather enigmatic, is the occurrence of 'infantile amnesia' – whereby most people cannot reliably remember information from before the age of about four years. It is not clear whether this phenomenon is due to i) biological processes, ii) state-dependent shifts in our mental state or 'set' from early childhood to later stages of life (which – as we saw in Chapter 3 – can prevent us from recalling information reliably), or to iii) some combination of these processes. One suggestion is that memories of earlier experiences before the age of 4 may well exist, but in a neural and/or psychological form which means that the individual can no longer access them as memories of specific experiences.

An anecdotal example of infantile amnesia and the seductive quality of childhood 'memories' was presented by the eminent Swiss developmental psychologist, Jean Piaget, who wrote: 'One of my first memories would date, if it were true, from my second year. I can still see, most clearly, the following scene, in which I believed until I was about fifteen. I was sitting in my pram, which my nurse was pushing in the Champs Élysées, when a man tried to kidnap me. I was held in by the strap fastened round me while my nurse bravely tried to stand between me and the thief. She received various scratches, and I can still see vaguely those on her face. Then a crowd gathered, a policeman with a short cloak and a white baton came up and the man took to his heels. I can still see the whole scene, and can even place it near the tube station. When I was about fifteen, my parents received a letter from my former nurse saying that she had been converted to the Salvation Army. She wanted to confess her past faults, and in particular to return the watch she had been given on this occasion. She had made up the whole story, faking the scratches. I, therefore, must have heard – as a child – the account of this story, which my parents believed, and projected it into the past in the form of a visual memory.'

Consistent with this account by Piaget, older children and adults may be able to remember early life events relatively well in general terms, but have problems specifying their origin because of the relative fragility in childhood of memory for context. So Piaget 'remembers' the event as it was told by the nurse (stating that 'I can still see, most clearly, the following scene . . . '), but at the same time he is apparently unable to appreciate fully (as a teenager) that the nurse was the source of this version of events – which, in reality, did not take place. Furthermore, early memories may be difficult to localize because they have been retrieved (and re-encoded) many times – and therefore cannot be reliably linked to a specific time or place. As previously discussed, context shifts (see Chapter 3) between the time of encoding and the time of retrieval may be especially relevant when adults are trying to retrieve events that were encoded during childhood. These possibilities are not mutually exclusive, but they are very difficult to investigate in a systematic, scientific manner.

As we saw in Chapter 4, we are all vulnerable to distortions in our memory. However, this may be especially the case when reflecting on events in our childhood, because of difficulties specifying a particular source and context. This has especially important implications when considering issues such as eyewitness testimony; the majority of evidence indicates that children are capable of providing accurate eyewitness testimony about personally significant events in their lives. However, the literature also indicates that, like adults, children's memory can be adversely influenced by false suggestions – but perhaps more so.

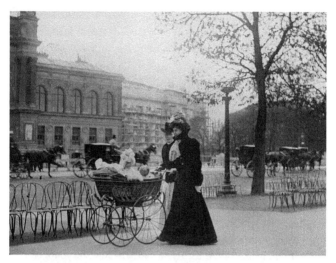

17. Older children and adults may be able to remember early life events relatively well in general terms, but have problems specifying their origin because of the relative fragility in childhood of memory for context. Piaget apparently 'remembered' the attempted kidnapping which allegedly occurred when he was in his pram in the Champs Élysées – even though he knew, logically, that the event had not taken place

Memory and ageing

An issue of relevance to all of us concerns our memory capacity as we age. Everyone experiences memory lapses, failure, and errors, but there may be a tendency in old people to attribute these automatically to the effect of ageing, rather than just to normal individual variability (with ageing being but an incidental factor). This important point was captured several centuries ago by the famous scholar, raconteur, and wit Samuel Johnson when he wrote:

There is a wicked inclination in most people to suppose an old man decayed in his intellects. If a young or middle-aged man, when leaving a company, does not recollect where he laid his hat, it is nothing; but if the same inattention is discovered in an old man, people will shrug up their shoulders, and say, 'His memory is going'.

Given the progressive increase in the average age of the population that is currently occurring (and will – most likely – continue to occur) in the majority of countries, it is important to identify what (if any) are the scientifically established memory changes that can be identified as a consequence of ageing. However, there are some significant methodological issues that need to be taken into consideration in this field. For example, if we compare the memory of 20-year-olds today with 70-year-olds today, there is a whole range of different factors that could explain differences in memory performance between these two groups of individuals – apart from the fact that the 20-year-olds are 50 years younger. For example, education and healthcare over the lifespan of the current 70-year-olds is likely to have been significantly inferior to that received by the current 20-year-olds. These extraneous – or confounding – factors could distort the outcome of studies into the effect of ageing on memory if we were to contrast the memory capacity of current 20-year-olds with the memory of current 70-year-olds.

Comparing the memory of current 20-year-olds with the memory of current 70-year-olds is an example of a *cross-sectional* experimental design. By contrast, in a *longitudinal* study the aim is to follow the same people across their lifespan from the age of 20 to 70, to see what changes in memory occur *within the same individuals* as people age. There are some advantages to this longitudinal method, in that we are comparing memory changes occurring in the same people. However, it has been noted that there is a tendency for a disproportionately large number of high-functioning people – that is, individuals with better preserved memory and other cognitive functions – to remain in a longitudinal study. (These people are sometimes called *super*

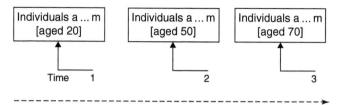

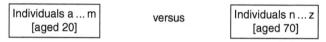

18. In a *longitudinal* study, we would follow the same people across their lifespan from the age of 20 to 70; whereas comparing the memory of current 20-year-olds with the memory of current 70-year-olds represents an example of a *cross-sectional* experimental design. There are pros and cons with each approach

controls or *super normals*.) In other words, what seems to happen in some longitudinal studies is that the people who are receiving positive feedback (related to their relatively well preserved functional capacity) from participation in a longitudinal study may continue to participate – whereas people who are struggling drop out. This may well result in an artificially positive impression of the effects of ageing. The other problem is – of course – finding someone (or, more likely, a team of people) who will be scientifically active for long enough to conduct longitudinal research, and analyse the data over a 50-year time period! In summary, both cross-sectional and longitudinal study designs have relative strengths and weaknesses.

Taking into consideration the findings of both cross-sectional and longitudinal studies, some consistent findings have emerged from studies into ageing and memory. In particular, it is noteworthy that there are parallels between the profile of memory capacity manifested by children and that of older adults.

Short-term memory seems to remain quite well preserved in older individuals, although tasks with more of a working memory element are often adversely affected by ageing (please refer back to Chapter 2 for this distinction). So where more cognitive work is involved (as distinct from more passive short-term storage) then deficits can be apparent. For example, age-related difficulties are likely to be more apparent when people are asked to repeat back a sequence of digits in reverse order, compared with when people are asked to repeat back a sequence of digits in the same order.

Performance on *explicit long-term memory* (i.e. memory with awareness of the memory experience; see Chapter 2) tasks typically declines significantly, especially on measures of free recall, although recognition holds up well with age. Recognition does seem to change qualitatively, though – by apparently becoming more familiarity based. So when recognition demands contextual memory (i.e. the more recollective component of recognition memory that we have considered previously; see Chapter 3), deficits do emerge with age. This may mean that older people (similar to children; see earlier in this chapter) are more susceptible to suggestion and bias in their memory. This could have important consequences in a real world context; for example, when older people are using their memory to make important decisions about matters such as their financial assets.

Implicit memory (i.e. memory without awareness, typically tested indirectly via the evaluation of changes in behaviour rather than recollection of the memory experience) seems to decline little with age. For example, an intriguing study of typing supporting this conclusion was conducted by Hill (1957), and involved Hill himself learning to type a passage of text aged 30 and then testing himself again aged 55 and 80! Hill's findings indicated (consistent with other similar studies) that not only does implicit memory mature relatively early in children, but it holds up well into old age.

There is little effect of ageing on *semantic memory*. In fact, this capacity seems to improve throughout life. For example, people's vocabulary and general knowledge usually increases as they get older (although they may experience greater problems accessing the relevant information; for example, with respect to the tip of the tongue phenomenon that we have considered in Chapters 2, 3, and 4). It has been suggested that the accumulation of information in semantic memory over the lifespan could explain why certain professions, in which the demands appear to load significantly on semantic knowledge, are occupied predominantly by older individuals (for example, high court judges, novelists, company chairpersons, admirals, professors, generals).

There is some evidence that age-related memory loss arises partly from relative degeneration in the frontal lobes of the brain, mediating the strategic and organizational aspects of memory. As mentioned earlier in this chapter, this portion of the brain appears to have developed disproportionately in humans relative to other species. As we noted, in children the emergence of meta-memory (i.e. one's awareness of one's memory abilities) also seems to be related to frontal lobe maturation, and there is evidence that age-related deterioration in meta-memory is associated with frontal lobe dysfunction. Prospective memory – or remembering to do something in the future – is another aspect of memory that has been linked to frontal brain functions; and, indeed, there is evidence that this capacity is adversely affected by ageing. The bottom line is that the frontal lobes seem to mature relatively late in life but start to deteriorate relatively early. Consistent with this, it has been suggested that the effects of frontal lobe dysfunction on memory can be detected in children and also in older people.

There is also evidence that age-related loss of memory capacity may be linked to a reduction in cognitive processing speed as we get older. Other proposals have suggested that age-related memory changes are caused by reduced inhibition, limitations in attention, and/or reduced contextual or environmental support.

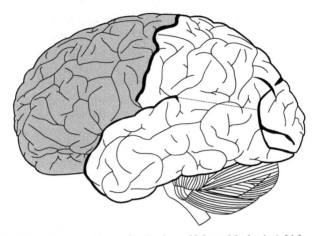

19. There is some evidence that the frontal lobes of the brain (which are disproportionately large in humans and are shown shaded on the left of this figure) mature relatively late in development and deteriorate relatively early, influencing the strategic and organizational aspects of memory

As with the 'frontal lobe hypothesis' of ageing, each of these accounts has limitations – but they have all generated interesting research questions.

One area of considerable interest is whether the changes in memory due to 'normal' ageing are necessarily hallmarks of further decline in brain capacity. An entity referred to as 'mild cognitive impairment' (MCI) has been defined as an intermediate category between normal ageing and clinical dementia. It has been proposed that MCI may be memory specific ('amnestic MCI') or may involve multiple cognitive domains ('multi-domain MCI'). It seems that a higher proportion of people diagnosed with MCI convert to full-blown dementia within a few years of the identification of this condition, but some people with MCI do not progress to dementia. Given the current 'demographic time bomb' of increasing numbers of elderly individuals living in most countries, at the present time there is considerable investment of resources directed at seeking to identify the factors that influence the progression from MCI to dementia. For example, recent evidence has indicated that factors such as exercise and a healthy diet (especially diets low in saturated fats and high in antioxidants) are not only healthy for the body, but they may well also help the brain to function well into old age.

In addition, mental exercise (such as crosswords, chess – and learning news skills such as information technology) may well be useful in maintaining neurological and psychological capacity. Moreover, research findings indicate that the brain maintains a degree of growth and repair capacity across the lifespan that can be induced by stimulating mental activity and exercise. This is an especially important consideration with respect to the optimal living environment for older individuals (for example, those who are admitted to residential homes due to physical frailty or cognitive difficulties). The hippocampus (part of the brain that appears to be centrally involved in memory consolidation, especially with respect to episodic memory – see Chapters 2 and 5) may be especially sensitive to neural regrowth and/or increased connectivity after mental stimulation or exercise.

With respect to age-related clinical disorders, memory dysfunction is typically an early hallmark of dementia. In particular, deficits in episodic memory and hippocampal functioning characterize the earliest stages of the most common form of dementia, senile dementia of the Alzheimer type. Episodic memory impairment can occur in relative isolation in the early stages of the illness. But later on in dementia, many other cognitive capacities can be affected – such as language, perception, and executive functions. It has also been suggested that the central executive of working memory (see Chapter 2) can be differentially impacted in Alzheimer's disease. Unlike people suffering from more selective forms of amnesia (see Chapter 5), people with Alzheimer's disease can be impaired on some tests of implicit as well as explicit memory, especially in the later stages of the illness – reflecting the

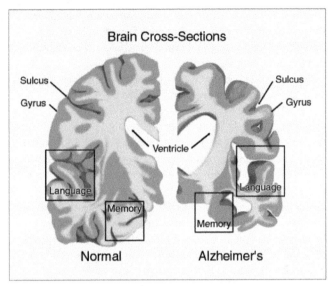

20. This figure shows shrinkage in the brain of someone with Alzheimer's disease (right) compared with a healthy elderly person (left). The parts of the brain subserving episodic memory are affected early in this illness

progression of the brain damage in this devastating illness. Another form of neurodegenerative illness has been termed semantic dementia. In contrast to Alzheimer's disease, this type of dementia involves a profound breakdown of semantic memory (see Chapter 2), such that people with this illness lose the ability to recognize familiar objects such as cups, tables, or cars.

At the moment, drug treatments that are available for dementia are symptomatic, treating the effects of the disease (such as reduced neurotransmission in the brain) rather than the fundamental causes of the illness. Furthermore, current treatments are not able to prevent the relentless progression of a neurodegenerative illness like Alzheimer's disease. This may change in the future, through techniques such as stem cell therapies or brain prostheses. In addition, cognitive rehabilitation techniques are effective in maximizing available memory capacity in people with neurodegenerative illness – helping to enhance self esteem and emotional status as well as functional capabilities (see Chapter 7).

As more diagnostic tests and possible treatments have become available, there is increasing interest in identifying measures of memory and cognition that are both sensitive and specific for MCI and dementia. If cognitive decline can be identified early enough, there is a greater chance that any degenerative process can be treated (or at least ameliorated) effectively.

Chapter 7
Improving memory

Many seminars, courses, and books are available in the commercial marketplace that claim to be able to significantly enhance our memory. This chapter will review the established objective, scientific evidence for techniques which may or may not be able to improve the functional efficiency of our memory. The focus will be on techniques such as mnemonics which may improve the efficiency of the 'software' of memory, but reference will also be made to possible future manipulation of the 'hardware' underpinning memory, whereby it may be possible in the future to use drugs, prosthetic devices and/or neural implants to attempt to correct problems in memory due to brain injury. We also consider mnemonists in this chapter (i.e. people with fantastic memory abilities) – particularly the person known as 'S'. People may often wish for a 'perfect memory', but the story of 'S' shows that being able to forget has distinct advantages.

Can you improve your memory?

The 'hardware'

At the present time, none of us can reliably improve the machinery underlying our memory, at least in terms of the biological 'hardware' involved. In scientific terms, there is currently no reliable way that the neural systems underlying memory can be systematically enhanced (although – of course – it is comparatively easy to damage these systems via head injury, alcohol and other forms of physical and chemical abuse).

There is some evidence that some agents (such as stimulants, e.g. nicotine or caffeine) can enhance our memory – often through improving our attention (and thereby improving our encoding of memory materials). However, these stimulant effects are only reliably observed when we are tired or our cognitive system is otherwise compromised. And if they make us *too* aroused, these stimulants may have counter-productive consequences. There have also been claims that certain 'smart drugs' and other neurochemical agents can improve the functioning of the neural components underlying memory. Such agents typically appear to act through enhancing chemical transmission or communication between brain cells. But, again, these substances are really only consistently helpful for some people with impaired memory due, for example, to brain damage or illness (such as dementia). By contrast, in healthy individuals (where the brain appears to be functioning at more or less its optimum capacity), the administering of such chemical agents does not really improve performance above this 'ceiling' level. A relatively crude analogy might be that of a car's engine: if you already have sufficient oil in the sump to lubricate the engine effectively, then adding more oil will not necessarily improve the functional efficiency of the engine and the transmission of power.

It might be possible to improve the 'neural hardware' underlying memory in the future – perhaps i) through genetic and neural manipulation and transplantation techniques, or ii) through the interfacing of carbon-based and silicon-based hardware. In the above, i) relates to putatively enhancing the substrate of our brain, whereas ii) relates to the use of prosthetic artificial devices. There have already been attempts to conduct both of these procedures in laboratory animals. However, these proposed techniques remain controversial. So at present, it seems that we can really only work with the neural hardware that we currently have available in our heads, and try to make sure that the 'software' running on those systems is working optimally. How do we do this?

The 'software'

What constitutes 'best practice' for remembering more?

When Ebbinghaus was learning his nonsense syllables, he found that there was a direct relationship between the number of learning trials and the amount of information retained (see Chapter 1). Ebbinghaus concluded that the amount learned was proportional to the time spent learning: other things being equal, if you doubled the amount of time spent learning, you would double the amount of information stored. This became known as the *total time hypothesis*, which is the basic relationship underlying the whole of the human learning literature. Yet, we have already seen that different types of memory encoding (such as 'deeper' versus 'shallower' levels of processing) produce differential levels of performance (Chapter 2). Moreover, we have seen in Chapter 1 how Ebbinghaus' memory techniques were in some ways artificial. So, despite the general relationship between the amount of practice and the amount remembered, there are other ways in which one can get a better return for time spent learning:

- The *distribution of practice effect* tells us that it is better to distribute learning trials across an extended period of time, rather than to mass trials together in a single block: 'little and often' is the key principal here. So cramming for an examination cannot replace solid, sustained revision.

- On a related theme, *errorless learning* is a flexible strategy in which a new item is initially tested after a short delay; then, as the item becomes better learned, the practice interval is gradually increased. The main aim is to test each item at the longest interval at which it can be reliably reproduced. This seems to work quite effectively as a learning technique. A beneficial by-product of errorless learning is that the motivation of the learner is sustained, because the rate of memory failure is kept at a low level.

- If you remember something for yourself (such as recalling the spelling of a word), this tends to strengthen the memory more effectively.

- Focusing attention on what you are learning is an effective approach. Victorian educators placed a lot of emphasis on repetition and rote learning; but repetition of information does not ensure that attention is being paid to the material (as we have seen previously in this book, nothing is likely to get into long-term memory unless you attend to it).

- Coding information both verbally and visually (i.e. creating a visual image of a verbal item), and creating 'mental maps' are often effective learning techniques. (The author Tony Buzan has produced a number of books and other publications describing the use of 'mental mapping' techniques. Please see Further reading on page 139.) The use of other types of mnemonic technique can also be very effective (see page 123).

- The way in which we process information is crucial. People seek meaning in information they are trying to remember, and if there is an absence of meaning, people try to impose their own meaning on the material (see Chapter 1, where we considered Bartlett's *War of the Ghosts* story). Building on this phenomenon, a general rule is that it often helps to relate new material to yourself and to your own circumstances as richly and elaborately as possible in the time available. And seeking to understand information that you are studying, rather than passively learning it, typically improves memory. (It seems that the processing of meaning typically links in more of our general knowledge, thereby semantically coding information more richly and improving subsequent memory performance.)

- Motivation to learn information is another important factor, although its effect may well be indirect (for example, if someone is highly motivated, this will influence the amount of time spent attending to the material to be learned – and this will typically improve the amount of learning taking place).

- There is a complex mutually reinforcing relationship between attention, interest, motivation, expertise and memory, so that the more knowledgeable you become in a particular field, the more interest you will have in it – and your knowledge and interest will reinforce each other in improving your memory for material in that field. An example of this might be the memory researcher, who finds it progressively easier to acquire and retain new findings in the field, the greater his or her expertise! The same principle applies to many walks of life; for example, the sales manager may be able to assimilate information about new products, building on his or her knowledge of products that have been sold in the marketplace over the past several decades.

In summary, improving memory performance requires application, initiative, and persistence, but there are also some reliable techniques that can help us. Furthermore, what we remember depends, in part, on how we were thinking, feeling, and acting at the time of the original experience (please refer to the state-dependent memory effects discussed in Chapter 3). This knowledge can allow us to develop strategies that help us modify what we remember.

We next consider in more detail some of the more significant factors influencing memorability of information.

Rehearsal

An early strategy often adopted by children is to repeat material over and over again 'in their heads'. The mere repetition of information, with no additional thought about meaning or associations, can help us to retain information for a few seconds, but it is generally a very poor method of learning for the longer term (see Chapter 2).

For example, Craik and Watkins asked participants to learn lists of words. In one condition, participants were encouraged to repeat the last few words in the list over and over again for some time before recall. Memory testing occurred immediately after the list had been presented. Participants recalled the repeated words well in the immediate test, but at the end of the experiment all of the different lists that had been presented were tested again. In the final test, the words that had been rehearsed repeatedly (and remembered better in the immediate test) were recalled no better than other words that had not been repeated by participants at all. The repetition was described as *maintenance rehearsal*. This kind of rehearsal apparently maintained information in memory temporarily, but did not improve longer-term memory.

In contrast to maintenance rehearsal, some participants in the Craik and Watkins study used *elaborative rehearsal*. Rather than passively repeating information in an effort to maintain its availability, in elaborative rehearsal the meaning of the information is considered by participants and this meaning is elaborated. Although both types of rehearsal can keep information available for a short time, it was found that recall after a delay is much better when the information has been rehearsed elaboratively than when it has merely been rehearsed in a maintenance fashion. It is as if elaborative rehearsal recodes the information so that it is retained more effectively (refer back to the 'levels of processing' framework cited in Chapter 2).

Expanding retrieval practice

Regardless of the type of rehearsal, later recall of information benefits from spaced *retrieval practice*, which involves trying to remember information over spaced time intervals. This method is sometimes called *expanding rehearsal* or *spaced retrieval*. This approach may be regarded as a technique for maximizing learning, with mental effort applied in an optimal manner. The underlying principle here is that memory is strengthened most when recall is attempted just before it becomes too difficult to accomplish. This time point is, of course, somewhat difficult to determine – such that reasonable estimates are typically made. It is interesting to reflect on how this principle dovetails with the principle of *errorless learning*, which is considered later in this chapter.

The fundamental principles underlying spaced retrieval are as follows. When we first encounter some information, it may be relatively fragile in terms of memorability. By successfully recalling the information correctly a short while after studying it, we are more likely to recall it again later – so we can allow a somewhat longer delay before our next successful retrieval effort. With each successful effort, the delay between each retrieval attempt can increase, and yet still lead to further successes.

The effectiveness of an expanding schedule for retrieval practice was demonstrated by Landauer and Bjork. These researchers read fictitious first and last names to participants, who were later asked to recall the fictitious last names when the fictitious first names were shown to them again. The tests were scheduled to explore a range of scenarios, including testing an *expanding schedule* – in which memory tests were at first introduced after a short delay, after which the interval was steadily increased. For the expanding schedule, the first test (for example, for the name *Jack Davies*) took place immediately, then the second test took place after three intervening items (for example, *Jack Davies*, then *Jim Taylor*, then *Bob Cooper* then *John Arnold*, followed by testing with the word Jack ------?), and then the third test occurred after ten further intervening items. In this study, Landauer and Bjork found that any retrieval practice was beneficial (relative to the control, unpractised condition), but that the greatest benefit was observed for this expanding schedule, which produced recall at approximately twice the level of unpractised items.

Expanding retrieval practice is an excellent strategy for students. It is relatively undemanding in terms of the effort and creativity required, and yet it can be applied to virtually any material.

The benefits of spaced study

A related concept concerns the advantages of spaced study. It may be natural to plunge intensively into trying to learn new information, but this strategy has been shown repeatedly to be misguided. The benefits of spacing study trials were observed by Ebbinghaus (see Chapter 1), who found that spreading his study sessions over three days approximately halved the amount of time required when recalling lists of nonsense syllables. In fact, two spaced presentations of material to be learned are often twice as effective as two concentrated, unspaced presentations.

Bahrick and Phelps demonstrated the robustness of the spaced study effect. They compared the performance of participants who had originally learned and then relearned Spanish vocabulary by testing them eight years after the teaching session. One group had originally learned and relearned the vocabulary with an interval between learning and relearning of 30 days, whereas the other group had learned and relearned the material on the same day. Eight years later, the participants who had learned and relearned the material with a 30-day interval showed a level of memory performance that was 250% higher than the same-day learning/relearning group!

Meaning and memory

Meaning has a major influence on memory, as we saw in Chapter 1 and elsewhere. Ebbinghaus argued that – if he was to discover the fundamental principles of memory – then he would need to study the learning of simple, systematically constructed materials. But while Ebbinghaus spent much of his time learning nonsense syllables, he nevertheless recognized that the study and retention of memory material could be influenced by its meaning.

As we saw in Chapter 1, Ebbinghaus created syllables by stringing together a consonant sound, a vowel sound, and a consonant sound. Some of these consonant-vowel-consonant trigrams comprised short words or meaningful parts of words, but most of these trigrams were relatively meaningless syllables. Ebbinghaus made lists of these syllables and learned them in order – often requiring many trials to learn them perfectly. In contrast to his relatively slow learning of these syllables, his acquisition of more meaningful materials such as poetry was considerably faster.

A further demonstration of the importance of meaning for the recall of very different material was provided by some relatively recent research conducted by Bower and colleagues into memory for *droodles* (i.e. simple line drawings of nonsense pictures). Some participants were given a meaning for each droodle (e.g. an elephant riding a monocycle). Bower and colleagues noted that the individuals who were given a meaning for each droodle were able to sketch the pictures from memory far better (70% correct) than participants who were not given these meanings (51% correct).

External aids

Nowadays we also have access to a number of artificial *external* memory aids, such as computers, personal digital assistants (PDAs), mobile phones, voice recorders, diaries, minutes, company reports, lecture notes, and so on. Perhaps the oldest example of an external memory aid is the knot in the handkerchief, which doesn't provide us with any information as such, but tells us that we need to search our memory system to recall an important piece of information.

External memory aids in the 21st century are sophisticated, and can work extremely well – until we don't or can't have them with

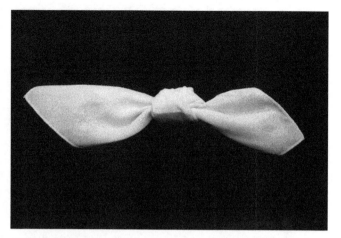

21. Perhaps the oldest example of an external memory aid is the knot in the handkerchief. This mnemonic doesn't provide us with any specific information, but tells us that we need to search our memory system to recall something important

us (for example, in some school or university examinations). If we want to improve our memory without having to rely on an artificial external aid, then (in addition to applying the principles outlined earlier in this chapter), we may wish to follow the example of people with so-called 'exceptional memory', who often use specific techniques called 'mnemonics'.

Mnemonics

A mnemonic is a way of organizing information to make it easier to remember – typically by using codes, visual imagery, or rhymes (sometimes in combination). Two well established methods are the 'method of loci' and 'pegwords'.

The method of loci

The oldest mnemonic method is the method of loci, taught from Classical times until the present day. The technique involves knowing a series of places or loci that are familiar yet distinct – students might use places around their school or university buildings. The first item to be remembered is imagined in the first of these places (i.e. by creating a mental image), the second item is imagined in the second place, and so on. The subsequent recall of this information then involves mentally revisiting the places and re-experiencing each of the images that were created earlier. Research has shown the technique to be highly effective, but its use can be limited by the relative unavailability of suitable locations and materials with which one can create images.

The origin of the technique is reputedly as follows. In about 500 BC, the Greek poet Simonides attended a celebration. Shortly after delivering a eulogy there, he was called away. This turned out to be a stroke of luck for him, because just after he left, the floor of the banqueting hall collapsed and several guests at the banquet were injured or killed. Many of the bodies from the tragedy were, allegedly, unrecognizable – making it impossible for relatives to identify the people in order to give them an appropriate burial. But Simonides found that he could quite easily remember where most of the guests had been seated at the time he left the banqueting hall, which made it much easier to identify the relevant individuals.

Based on this experience, Simonides was said to have devised a general mnemonic technique. The method involved visualizing a room or building in great detail, and then imagining various to-be-remembered objects or pieces of information placed in particular locations. Whenever Simonides needed to remember what these items were, he would imagine himself walking through the room or building and 'picking up' those items, i.e. collecting those specific pieces of information. This system of memorizing became popular with Classical orators like Cicero, who had to remember very long sequences of text for their orations. Indeed, it is still used today (for example, by people giving speeches at weddings – where it is often important to remember a sequence of

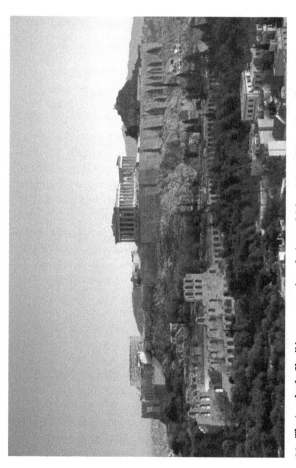

22. The 'method of loci' is a mnemonic technique which originated in ancient Greece. The method involves visualizing a room or building in great detail, and then imagining various to-be-remembered objects or pieces of information placed in particular locations within that building or room

items in a particular order). The technique seems to work particularly well with concrete words, such as the names of objects, which can be 'placed' in a particular location. But it can also work with abstract words, such as 'truth', 'hope', and so on – provided the person can generate a representative image of the abstract concept and locate it appropriately.

Pegwords

The method of loci has since been elaborated into the more flexible *pegword* system, using a phonetic mnemonic in the construction of the pegwords: '1 is a bun, 2 is a shoe, 3 is a tree, 4 is a door, 5 is a hive, 6 is sticks, 7 is heaven, 8 is a gate, 9 is wine, 10 is a hen'. Suppose you need to remember a shopping list, and the first word in your list is 'birthday card'. Using pegwords, you link this with the image associated with number 1, bun. So you might create a visual image of a bun sitting on top of a birthday card. If the second word is 'orange juice', you might think of juice being poured into shoe – generally speaking, the more bizarre the image, the better this technique seems to work. Furthermore, this method is particularly useful when one needs to remember things in a specific sequence (such as a series of road names forming a particular route).

As with the method of loci, this technique can be used for a wide range of materials that need to be remembered – one simply needs to link each item in the sequence to each of the pegwords, by making a particularly evocative and memorable association. *Pegword mnemonics* allow a much more flexible use of the imagery mnemonic than the method of loci and can be dramatically effective. Indeed, they form the basis of most professional memory improvement techniques. The pegs provide easily accessed memory cues, while the use of imagery links the cue and the item to be remembered through robust visuo-spatial associations.

So, in this technique easily imagined pegwords replace the places of the method of loci. Although the technique remains based on visual imagery, using the pegword technique we might learn words to represent each of the numbers from 1 to 100. The technique is designed so that the pegwords themselves are easily learned – because they are constructed according to a few simple rhyming rules which permit numbers to be strongly associated with the pegwords.

Other imagery mnemonics using the pegword technique have been developed. For example, Morris, Jones, and Hampson evaluated a technique that was recommended by several professional memory performers. To remember a name, it first had to be converted into some easy-to-image pegword form. For example, the name Gordon could be converted into a 'garden'. Then a garden would be imagined growing on some prominent feature of the person's face to link the pegword cue (i.e. the word 'garden') and the item to be remembered (i.e. the name of the person). By this method, the pegword cue 'garden' could be deciphered into 'Gordon' to produce the correct name on presentation of the person's face. Morris, Jones, and Hampson found that this mnemonic produced an overall 80% improvement in the learning of names.

Similar techniques have been extended to language learning, such as the *Linkword system* (developed extensively by Gruneberg). By this technique, foreign words are converted into some similar sounding English word that can be easily imaged. An evocative mental image is then formed to link the image with the actual meaning of the foreign word. So, for example, the French for rabbit is *lapin* – so one might imagine a rabbit sitting in someone's lap.

In a recent book, Wilding and Valentine describe studies of memory champions and other memory experts, many of whom have discovered for themselves the value of mental imagery as a memory improvement technique. The use of imagery is not essential for memory improvement, but it represents a powerful method whereby material that is superficially relatively meaningless and disconnected can be made more meaningful and connected – and therefore easier to remember.

Verbal mnemonics

Although classical mnemonics relied mainly on visual imagery (such as the method of loci), in later times verbal mnemonics were developed. For example, a simple way of connecting words from a list is to compose a story. Research has shown that asking people to make up a story that links together a list of words makes later recall of those words much better. In addition, many students are familiar with rhymes such as '30 days hath September, April, June and November...', where rhythm and rhymes provide structures that aid recall.

Mnemonics using verbal materials tend to fall into one of two categories: using either a *reduction code* or an *elaboration code*. A reduction code reduces the amount of information (for example, to remember certain rules of trigonometry, my father was taught at school to use the nonsense word *SOHCAHTOA*), whereas an elaboration code increases or meaningfully recodes the same information (to learn the same trigonometric relationships, I was taught at school to use the expression *Some Old Horses Chew Apples Heartily Throughout Old Age*). Another example of an elaboration code is the first-letter mnemonic *Richard Of York Gave Battle In Vain*, which helps us to remember the colours of the rainbow by matching the first letter of each word (Red, Orange, Yellow, Green, Blue, Indigo, Violet).

For both elaboration and reduction codes, the coding technique produces information that is easier to remember than the original source material, because the coded information is typically more meaningful to the user than the original source information. Such techniques have been used to remember, for example, dates in history. By assigning numbers to the letters of the alphabet, if one is having trouble remembering a specific date, such as 1815 for the

Battle of Waterloo, this could instead be re-coded as AHAE. Although this is a nonsense word, it could be more meaningful to the person concerned than the number itself (for example, it could be used to create an acronym, such as 'An Historic Attack (in) Europe'). Of course, as with every mnemonic, the time and energy invested in deriving and applying the mnemonic has to be weighed against the potential added value that the mnemonic contributes in remembering.

Reduction codes and elaboration codes can be used together. For example, as a medical student I was taught to remember the cranial nerves via a code which first reduced the first letter of each of the cranial nerves (O, O, O, T, T, A, F, A, G, V, A, H), and then transformed these letter via an elaboration code into a bawdy (and very memorable!) verse. As I write this book almost twenty five years later, I can still remember the verse, even if I may struggle a little to convert back from the verse to the original source information (i.e. the names of the twelve cranial nerves). This example illustrates the enduring quality of some mnemonics, but also indicates one potential problem, i.e. when the 'mnemonic code' becomes disassociated from the source material. So some mnemonics may work best when the source material is readily accessible, but merely needs to be structured or sequenced appropriately.

Other forms of well-learned information can also be used to supplement memory for facts or stimuli. For example, musical people may find that by setting particular words to a well known tune, memory for those words can be enhanced. This technique has been used by students for remembering complex sequences (such as biochemical pathways) and for retaining elaborate structural and conceptual frameworks (such as the inter-relationships of different neuroanatomical structures). And people who are fascinated by numbers sometimes find that strings of digits have rich personal associations. These associations can then be stored in long-term memory, making it easier to remember long strings of digits in a series of 'chunks', rather than as individual digits (assuming, of course, that the to-be-remembered digit strings can be related to the number 'chunks' that are already stored in long-term memory). For example, someone interested in numbers or mathematics may have committed to memory that the first four digits of *pi* are 3.142, and they may then be able to use this information to help them to code other numbers for subsequent remembering.

Remembering names

As we have seen throughout this book, meaning plays a major role in determining what we can remember. Consider the case of remembering names. People who feel they have a bad memory commonly complain that they find names especially difficult to remember. In fact, people are generally poor at dealing with a new name. When introduced to a new person, our minds are usually otherwise occupied (for example, by a parallel conversation), and so we often fail to attend to that person's name. Then we most likely do not use or try to think of the person's name until much later, by which time memory often fails. We can improve our memory for people's names by paying full attention and saying that person's name back to them when we first are introduced.

But there is more to the problem of remembering names than merely not paying attention to and not using someone's name until much later. Cohen and Faulkner presented participants with information about fictitious people: their names, the places they came from, their occupations, and hobbies. The participants remembered all the other attributes of these fictitious people better than their names. Why? It would seem that this is not simply because names are unfamiliar words, because many names are also common nouns (e.g. Potter, Baker, Weaver, Cook). Systematic research studies have been conducted in which people studied the same set of words – but sometimes the words were presented as names, and other times as occupations. Notably, the same words were remembered much better when they were presented as occupations rather than as names. So, it is apparently easier to learn that someone is a carpenter than that they are named Mr Carpenter!

Nevertheless, it seems that names that are also real words do have an advantage (in terms of their probability of being remembered) over 'non-word' names. The lack of meaningful (i.e. semantic) associations to some names may be part of the explanation for why they are harder to learn. Cohen has shown that meaningful words presented as names (e.g. Baker) are better remembered than names which are less meaningful (such as Snodgrass). But in the 21st century names are often treated as being meaningless – think for a second how it sometimes comes as a surprise when we recognize that they are also occupations or objects (for example, the names of the recent political leaders, Thatcher and Bush). Indeed, it is known that attending to the meaning of someone's name can improve memory for this name, especially when this is combined with practice in recalling them. Furthermore, if we can form associations between someone's appearance and their name, then we can improve our memory for that person's name – especially if we are able to form a salient visual image. So, if we meet someone called Jack who looks like an actor we know called Jack, or if we meet someone called Taylor who is wearing fine clothes, then we may well be able to use these associations to improve our memory for that person's name.

Reflecting on our own learning

Metamemory refers to the understanding that we have of our own memory. How accurate are we at judging how well we have learned something? This is an important consideration – because if we can adequately judge how well (or poorly) we have learned material, we can apply this knowledge to inform our subsequent study plans, spending additional time on material that is less well learned. What does the objective evidence indicate? If a judgement is made soon after studying material, it seems that we are comparatively poor at predicting our later memory performance. On the other hand, when the judgement is made after a delay, it seems that we are relatively better at making this judgement. Some additional research suggests that, in some learning situations, people are more likely to schedule their study time with emphasis on areas that they know well or find particularly interesting – but neglecting areas that need work. This finding indicates that we need to discipline ourselves to structure our time systematically across the topics that we are required to assimilate if we are to learn effectively.

The man with a perfect memory

Happiness is nothing more than good health and a bad memory.

Albert Schweitzer

People often wish for a 'perfect memory'. But the following story shows that being 'able' to forget has distinct advantages. Shereshevskii (or 'S'), whose story is reported in Luria's book *The Mind of a Mnemonist*, had a truly remarkable memory, which relied very heavily on imagery. He also seemed to manifest a particular phenomenon called *synaesthesia*, whereby certain stimuli provoke unusual sensory experiences. To a person with this condition, hearing a particular sound might evoke a specific smell, or seeing a certain number might evoke a particular colour.

'S' was first discovered when, as a journalist, his editor noticed that he was exceptionally good at remembering instructions that he was given before he investigated a story. Indeed, 'S' appeared to manifest close to perfect recall of even apparently meaningless information. However complex the briefing he received, it seemed that he never had to take notes, and he could repeat anything that was said to him almost word for word. 'S' took this ability for granted, but his editor persuaded him to see a psychologist, A. R. Luria, for tests. Luria set a series of increasingly complex memory tasks, including lists of more than 100 digits, long strings of nonsense syllables, poetry in unknown languages, complex figures and elaborate scientific formulae. Not only could 'S' repeat this material back perfectly, but he could also perform tasks such as repeating the information back in reverse order. He could even recall the information several years later.

The secret of 'S's' exceptional memory seems to be that he was able to create a wealth of evocative visual and other sensory associations without too much effort, probably related to his synaesthesia. This meant that even information that appeared dry and dull to other people created a vivid multimodal sensory experience for 'S' – not only in visual terms but also, for example, in terms of sound, touch, and smell. So 'S' could encode and store any piece of information in a very rich and elaborate way.

One may imagine that it would be wonderful to have an almost perfect memory – as 'S' did. But in fact, forgetting is generally quite adaptive, in that (as a general rule) we tend to remember those things that are important to us, while those things that are less important to us tend to fade. So, generally speaking, our memory tends to work like a sieve or filtering mechanism to ensure that we don't remember absolutely everything. By contrast, 'S' tended to remember almost everything, and his life became quite miserable. The main problem for 'S' seemed to be that new information (such as idle talk from other people) set off an uncontrollable train of distracting memory associations for him. Eventually, 'S' could not even hold a conversation, let alone function as a journalist.

However, 'S' did become a professional mnemonist, giving demonstrations of his extraordinary skills on stage – so he used his ability to earn his living. But he had tremendous difficulty forgetting some of the abstract information that he reproduced during these performances, finding that his memory became more and more cluttered with all sorts of useless information that he didn't need, and would rather forget.

Advice when studying for an examination or test

Memory depends very much on the perspicuity, regularity, and order of our thoughts. Many complain of the want of memory, when the defect is in the judgment; and others, by grasping at all, retain nothing.

Thomas Fuller

- Select a working environment that doesn't have too many distractions, so you can focus on the target information rather than on distractors that may be occurring in the environment. (Recall the importance of paying attention and appropriately encoding target materials for subsequent memory performance – as discussed earlier in this chapter.) This point notwithstanding, people often find that music can assist in creating a relaxed environment that is suitable for study, although (for reasons probably related to distraction) a more familiar piece of music is likely to be more helpful in this respect than a novel piece. A related point is to try to encode the information as actively as possible – for example, when reading a textbook, imagine yourself questioning the author of the piece. Try to relate what is being said to what you already know.

- Think about the interrelationships between different concepts, facts and principles in the field that you are studying (this will not only help you when you are trying to learn the material in preparation for an examination, but it will often also help you in answering the questions set during the exam itself).

- Think broadly about the topics you are studying and try to imagine their application to problems in your everyday life, i.e. problems you have encountered personally.

- Relate new material to yourself and your own interests as richly and elaborately as possible. You are then likely to make a much better job of reproducing that information in an examination context.

- Related to the last point: try to learn *actively* rather than *passively*. It is often said that the best way to learn a subject is to teach it, because to convey the information to someone else, you must be able to reproduce it – not just in a passive way, but also with understanding. In other words, don't move on in your study as soon as you can recognize the correct answer, but only when you can reproduce this answer spontaneously without being prompted, and you can explain the material comprehensibly to yourself or to someone else. (Study groups formed with other students can be useful in this respect.)

- Organization of information helps in two ways: i) by structuring what is being learned, so that recalling a fragment of that information may well recall the whole, and because ii) by relating newly learned material to one's existing knowledge structure, it is easier to comprehend new material.

- Practice is also important – you can't completely escape the effects of the 'total time hypothesis', which states that (other things being equal) the amount you learn depends on the amount you practise. This applies whether you are learning facts, theories, movements in a dance sequence, or a foreign language. However, as we saw earlier in this chapter, massing all your practice together into a marathon learning session (such as cramming for an examination) is not an efficient way of learning – little and often is a much better learning strategy (using techniques such as spaced retrieval).

- Use those times in your life when there's an unoccupied interval to good effect (for instance, if you are waiting for a bus and you have some study material to remember, use that time effectively). Keep a selection of notes on cards, or use your laptop, PDA or mobile phone to jot down notes, to create associations and mental maps, and to refresh your memory of the to-be-remembered material.

- Based on their research findings, Bransford and colleagues have laid great emphasis on 'transfer appropriate processes' or 'encoding specificity' (see Chapter 3). This principle states that what is important about a learning task is how it 'transfers' knowledge to the testing situation. By this view, people should try to engage in activities during learning which mimic what they will need to do in a test or examination situation – in order to optimize subsequent memory performance.

- On a related note, do not study when tired, and try to undertake your revision as much as possible when you are in a similar type of physical and emotional context as you are likely to be in at the time of the examination (e.g. seated at a simple table or desk). And you will attend to information better and encode stimuli more richly when you are alert rather than fatigued.

- Related to consistency in physical and emotional context, we saw in Chapter 3 how a change of context can adversely affect recall. Indeed, sometimes trying mentally to reconstruct the context in which one learned information (e.g. through imagery) can be useful for enhancing subsequent recall.

- Last but not least, consider using visual imagery and mnemonic techniques (such as those outlined in this chapter) to enhance your memory.

- The general message here is that good memory demands a high level of attention, motivation, and organization, and this in turn depends upon personal interest.

Final thoughts

Memory plays a critical role in many aspects of our daily existence. Indeed, without memory many other important capacities (such as language, the identification of familiar objects, or the maintenance of social relationships) would not be possible. It should be apparent after reading this book that memory represents a collection of abilities rather than a unitary capacity (as might be implied by an unfortunate tendency to refer to our memory in the singular in everyday speech). Moreover, memory is not a passive receptacle, nor is it necessarily a truthful recording of events in our lives. It is an *active* and *selective* process, with both strengths and weaknesses – which often represent the opposite sides of the same coin. Human memory is prone to a number of errors, many of which we have considered in this book. At the same time, our memory tends to record important events in our lives. So, we may propose the following seven defining features of memory:

1. Memory is important to people; it plays a role in comprehension, learning, social relationships, and in many other aspects of life.

2. Memory for a past event or information is indicated whenever a past event or information influences someone's thoughts, feelings, or behaviour at some later time. (The person need not be aware of any memory for the past event, and might not even have been aware of the event when it occurred; the intention to remember is also unnecessary.)

3. Memory is observed through free recall, cued recall, recognition, familiarity, and other behavioural changes such as priming and our physical actions.

4. Memory seems to involve more than just one system or type of process, as there is evidence that different sorts of memories can be influenced differently by specific manipulations or variables.

5. Memory is difficult to study – in that it must be inferred from observable behaviour.

6. Memory is not a veridical copy of a past event – events are constructed by people as they occur; remembering involves the re-construction of the event or information.

7. Psychologists have improved our understanding of many variables that influence memory, but there is still much to learn. Nevertheless, we can each be wiser users of our own memory by using effective mnemonic strategies and directing our efforts appropriately to help us learn and remember information.

Further reading

Introductory texts

Alan D. Baddeley, *Essentials of Human Memory* (Psychology Press, 1999). A fully referenced yet accessible overview of memory for the general reader, written by an international expert in the field. Each chapter contains suggestions for Further reading.

Tony Buzan, *Use Your Memory* (BBC Consumer Publishing, 2003). Provides an overview of mnemonic techniques from one of the most popular writers in the field who has published a range of other related texts.

Michael W. Eysenck and Mark T. Keane, *Cognitive Psychology: A Student's Handbook* (Psychology Press, 2005). Provides an overview of the core psychological processes which interface with, and impact upon, memory capacity – and which are themselves influenced by the operating characteristics of human memory (including attention, language, decision-making, and reasoning).

Daniel L. Schacter, *The Seven Sins of Memory* (Houghton Mifflin, 2001). Discusses the pros and cons of human memory in a lucid, informative, and entertaining manner.

More advanced texts

Gérard Emilien, Cécile Durlach, Elena Antoniadis, Martial Van der Linden, and Jean-Marie Maloteaux, *Memory: Neuropsychological, Imaging and Psychopharmacological Perspectives* (Psychology Press, 2003). Considers the biological processes that mediate and impact upon memory function, including the effects of brain injury and drugs, together with insights gained from neuro-imaging studies.

Jonathan K. Foster and Marko Jelicic, *Memory: Systems, Process or Function?* (Oxford University Press, 1999). Considers the central debate of how human memory should be conceptualized in theoretical and practical terms.

Endel Tulving and Fergus I. M. Craik (eds.), *The Oxford Handbook of Memory* (Oxford University Press, 2000). A *magnum opus* reviewing the field of memory research, with individual chapters written by the world's leading memory scientists.

Index

Memory

ONLINE
CATALOGUE
A Very Short Introduction

Our online catalogue is designed to make it easy to find your ideal Very Short Introduction. View the entire collection by subject area, watch author videos, read sample chapters, and download reading guides.

SOCIAL MEDIA
Very Short Introduction

Join our community
www.oup.com/vsi

- Join us online at the official Very Short Introductions **Facebook** page.
- Access the thoughts and musings of our authors with our online **blog**.
- Sign up for our monthly **e-newsletter** to receive information on all new titles publishing that month.
- Browse the full range of Very Short Introductions online.
- Read **extracts** from the Introductions for free.
- Visit our library of **Reading Guides**. These guides, written by our expert authors will help you to question again, why you think what you think.
- If you are a teacher or lecturer you can order inspection copies quickly and simply via our website.